Personality And The Body

By J.H. Effenberg, Ph.D.

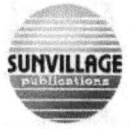

www.sunvillagepublications.com

Personality And The Body
By J.H. Effenberg, Ph.D.

Copyright © 2010

No part of this publication may be reproduced, stored in a retrieval
system or transmitted in any form or by any means, electronic,
mechanical, photocopying, recording or otherwise, without prior written
permission from the publisher.

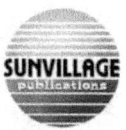

www.sunvillagepublications.com

Cover design by www.WebCopyAlchemy.com

PERSONALITY AND THE BODY

"Man must build his culture about the complete human personality. Whatever nourishes the personality—humanizes it—refines it—deepens it—intensifies its aptitudes, and broadens its field of action—is good.

"Whatever limits it—thwarts it—limits its capacity for human co-operation and communion—must be counted bad."

LEWIS MUMFORD

Dedicated with warmest affection

To my wife, Emmy Hoil Effenberg, whose assistance and inspiration were a great help in writing this book;

To our children, Steve, Agnes, Irme, Johnny, Joyce, Herbert, and Christol, in hopeful expectation; and

To the wonderful men and women of this generation who earnestly strive to perfect their personalities.

J. H. E.

ABOUT THE AUTHOR

DR. J. H. EFFENBERG was born in Dresden, capital of Saxony. He received his main education in Germany, afterward taking graduate studies in the Far East and the United States. He attended five universities and other institutes of learning, including the universities of Halle, Wittenberg, and Friedrich Wilhelm, of Breslau. He received his mission training at the Mission Seminary of Friedensau, in Germany, and at the Oriental Language Institute, in Shanghai, he studied in the Chinese language for three and a half years. He holds several degrees, among them a doctorate in psychology, and he is a certified grapho-analyst.

Dr. Effenberg held a pastorate for many years, eight years in Germany and twenty-four years in China, and conducted missions in religion and physical and mental health.

During World War I, as noncombatant, he served as Hospital Master in the German Army, and in the Turkish Army as a Medical Corps officer.

During World War II he served as superintendent of the Wuchan Sanitarium and Hospital in Central China.

After World War I, he organized the SDA Medical Cadet work in Germany, and also became the first Medical Cadet director for this work in China. In acknowledgment and recognition of this work, the National Red Cross Executive Council of China bestowed upon him the rank of "Red Cross General."

As superintendent of missions in China, Dr. Effenberg worked with, and under the direction of, the famous "China doctor," Dr. Harry Willis Miller. Among his many friends he counted such notable Moslem leaders as Governor Ma Lin, Ma Bu Fang, and others. For work done, especially during World War II, he received letters of appreciation from notable places, also from the headquarters of Generalissimo Chiang Kai-shek,

President of Free China. He values highly a handwritten letter of gratitude from the Honorable Chen Cheng, presently Vice President of Free China.

In his extensive travels in China and its borderlands, Dr. Effenberg visited many lamaseries in Tibet and Mongolia, and conversed with many high-ranking and learned lamas and "living Buddhas."

PREFACE

THE OLD English jester was a playful joker who often hid deep truths in his jokes. The story is told of an English nobleman who gave his jester a wand, saying: "Jester, keep this until you find a greater fool than yourself." Laughingly the jester accepted the wand and flourished it on festive occasions.

One day, the nobleman lay dying. He called the jester to his bedside, and the following conversation took place.

Nobleman: I am going on a long journey.

Jester: Where to?

Nobleman: I don't know.

Jester: How long will you be gone?

Nobleman: I shall be gone forever.

Jester: What provision have you made for your trip?

Nobleman: None at all.

Jester: Then take this with you. (He pressed the wand into the nobleman's hand.) I have found the one fool greater than I.

The moral of the story is that all those who fail to realize the purpose of life, who don't build for the future, who are found unprepared for that last journey everyone has to take, run a foolish risk.

There is only one thing man can take with him into the life hereafter, and that is a personality developed and perfected after the likeness of his Creator.

The greatest literary work ever written dealing with human personality is the Holy Scriptures. I am a firm believer in the Holy Scriptures as God's inspired word. I can find no better guide for "personality engineering." Therefore I shall make no apologies for my frequent references to this source throughout this book. "I have set the Lord always before me" (Ps. 16:8). "Thou wilt show me the path of life" (Ps. 16:11). This study is a long one, and I realize I risk boring the reader with the many "don'ts" and prohibitions. But the positive side, if practiced and followed, will bring sure blessings, and a practical foundation for a real personality.

Grateful acknowledgments are made to A. W. Truman, M.D., F.A.C.S., F.I.C.S., Robert E. Maxson, Eva E. Maxson, and Ethel Davis, who read the original draft of the manuscript of this book and made valuable critical comments and suggestions. The contents, however, are the full responsibility of the author.

This book is really the first part of a three-part study on how to become an effective personality. Here we discuss the body. The second and third parts discuss the soul and the spirit, respectively. Although each volume is complete in itself, to receive the full benefit a study of all three is imperative.

J. H. E.

CONTENTS

PERSONALITY AND THE BODY

I will instruct thee
and teach thee in the
way
which thou shalt go:

I will guide thee
with mine eye.

The Great "I AM"

PSALM 32:8
Exodus 3:14)

1. WHO IS RESPONSIBLE?

THE WHOLE reveals the condition of its parts, and the parts are not better than the whole, and vice versa. A chain at its best is never stronger than its weakest link. In using this yardstick to measure society today—turbulent world affairs, ever growing lawlessness, mounting wickedness, juvenile delinquency, terrifying preparations for war and mutual destruction—we get clear evidence that it is badly overbalanced with negative character traits.

Covetousness, arrogance, self-love, egoism, anger, temper, hate, strife, evil, murder, corruption, and malignity are rampant and violent. Similar language was used by Paul the Apostle when in a vision about the end of the time he saw and described the condition of the Human Society.

"Mark this," said he, "there are hard times coming in the last days. For men will be selfish—fond of money—boastful-haughty—abusive—disobedient to their parents—ungrateful—irrev-erent—callous—relentless—scurrilous—reckless and conceited, preferring pleasure to God." (I Tim. 3:1-4, Moffat.) If Paul were alive today, he would say the same thing except for one change— what he then put in the future tense, he would put in the present tense today.

Who is responsible for this state of society, and the conditions we have today? The weakness of the whole is in the weakness of its parts. If I want to better the world, I have to start with me—my family, my community, my country. If it is true that a chain is never stronger than its weakest link, what of a country? Can a country be stronger than its citizens? Remember, it is not its savage strength but its moral strength that makes a country strong and lasting. "The true grandeur of humanity is in moral elevation, sustained, enlightened, and decorated by the intellect of man," says C. Sumner. All the great countries that relied on their savage strength, like Babylon, Medio-Persia, Greece, and Rome: where are they? In oblivion; gone and forgotten.

The weakness shown by the whole today is the weakness of its parts, a sure cry for personality engineering. Let us learn, and pray from the bottom of our hearts, that beautiful prayer of St. Francis of Assisi:

> Lord, make me an instrument of peace—
> where there is hatred, let me show love;
> where there is injury, pardon;
> where there is doubt, faith;
> where there is despair, hope;
> where there is darkness, light;
> where there is sadness, joy.
>
> O Divine Father, grant that I may not so much seek
> to be consoled as to console;
> to be understood as to understand;
> to be loved as to love;
> for it is by giving that we receive;
> it is in pardoning that we are pardoned;
> it is by dying that we are born to eternal life.

Who is responsible? Not I, you may reply. It's not my fault, you may utter with emphasis. I am what I am by inheritance. I cannot help it. I talk, I walk, I act the way I am built.

No, my friend, authorities on heredity inform us that character and personality are not inheritable. We may inherit a favorable disposition for certain habits that form character traits, but not the habits or the traits themselves. We cannot inherit education; we have to acquire it by studying. We cannot inherit muscles; we have to develop them by constant use. Equally, we cannot inherit habits and traits, which form our character and personality. They must be built, be formed by constant repetition.

We are not personalities, when born into this world; neither are we psychological Melchizedeks, perfect, full grown, without father and mother. Personality is not a natural endowment bestowed equally upon everybody. It is not a gift of the Creator, which He has distributed to just a chosen few.

Personality is a product that must be unfolded, developed, and perfected during the life span of each individual. True, each of us is born into this world under a different set of circumstances, a different environment, and a different station in life, but we all have the great privilege and the symphonic task to develop, harmonize, and perfect our physical, intellectual, and spiritual parts into a personality reflecting the likeness of our wonderful Creator.

When we were born we were not charged with the debts and plunderings of our parents and ancestors. No, Nature kindly opened a new book for us and gave us a clear account sheet, with the opportunity to start afresh "to build our own personality—to write our own story." Therefore, as E. G. White says:

Be not satisfied with reaching a low standard. We are not what we might be, or what it is God's will that we should be.

Never think that you have learned enough, and that you may now relax your efforts. Your education should continue during your lifetime. Every day you should be learning, and putting to practical use the knowledge gained.

Remember that in whatever position you may serve, you are revealing motive, developing character.

Who is responsible? Let us close with the fitting words of Henley's poem:

> It matters not how strait the gate,
> How charged with punishments the scroll,
> I am the master of my fate;
> I am the captain of my soul.

2. THE WORTH OF PERSONALITY

THE HIGHEST, most admirable aspiration of any person is a forceful and charming personality. It will be interesting, delightful, and rewarding to study how to become a personality, and you may cherish such a study for the rest of your life. It also will be the greatest, deepest, and most complex problem you have ever had to solve, because there is none vaster in scope. But when solved satisfactorily, its recompense is incalculably greater and more gratifying than anything else.

THE SUPREME ELEMENT

In the relationship of people in the business world and in social life, personality, not money or possessions, is the foremost and supreme element.

The following incident happened in one of the highest courts of this country. It will serve to illustrate the foregoing statement. During a Congressional investigation of credit, the late financier J. P. Morgan was called to the witness stand by Attorney Untermyer, who interrogated him as follows.

Q. Mr. Morgan, is credit not based upon money?

A. No, sir, it has no relationship. I know lots of men, business men, too, who can borrow any amount, and whose credit is unquestionable.

Q. Is that not because it is believed that they have money back of them?

A. No, sir, it is because people believe in the man.

Q. And this is regardless of whether he has financial backing at all?

A. It is very often.

Q. And he might not be worth anything?

A. He might not have anything. I have known a man to come

to my office, and I have given him a check for a million dollars, and knew he had not a cent in the world.

Q. There are not many of them?

A. Yes, sir, a good many.

Q. Are not commercial credits based upon possessions or properties?

A. No, sir, the first and foremost is *character and personality.*

Yes, personal force and character are the only investments worth anything. The man with a personality is the trusted employee, the responsible executive, the leader in every field of endeavor, commercial, social, and spiritual. He is the man of distinction. If a man puts forth all the effort necessary to develop personality, the result will pay him great dividends.

PERSONALITY   DEFINED

What is "personality"? What does this term indicate? What is its full meaning? The Encyclopaedia Britannica gives the following definitions:

> PERSON: an individual, a human being including body and mind.
> PERSONALITY: that which constitutes a person, plus that which
>   distinguishes and characterizes a person.

Basecus' Word Bank defines it thus:

> *PERSONALITY:* the whole; all the characteristics of a person.

Another writer gives this definition:

> PERSONALITY is the distinctive moral make-up of a person,
>   which dominates all his thinking, feeling and action.

But we find the best, clearest, and most complete definition in the Holy Scriptures (I Thess. 5:23, King James version):

> The very God of peace sanctify you wholly; and I pray God your
>   whole spirit and soul and body be preserved blameless . . .

In the 1961 Oxford University translation this reads:

> The very God of peace make you holy in every part, and
> keep you sound in spirit, soul and body.

Here it is set clearly before us: we are a trinity. Our personality is
constructed of three parts, distinguished as:

> SPIRIT: the spiritual part—the highest division.
> SOUL: the intellectual part—the innermost kernel. BODY:
> the physical part—the outside shell.

Here is the outline and direction for our study: How to Become a
Personality. Close attention should be paid and great care must be
given to each single part, to the physical, mental, and spiritual
system. If we neglect to care for and develop our own trinity by
neglecting just one part, we will soon become useless to ourselves
and also to the rest of the world. Perfecting our personality will
then be impossible, because the whole consists of *all* its parts.

3. THE GREAT DIVERSITY

> The world is so full of a number of things,
> I'm sure we should all be as happy as kings.
>   ROBERT LOUIS STEVENSON

ONE OF THE greatest wonders in the universe is the diversity of
things. There are billions of leaves on the trees, and no two are
alike. There are billions of stars in the heavens, and no two are the
same. There are billions of snowflakes, of flowers, of insects, and
billions upon billions of other things, yet each one is different
from all the others. There are more than two billion people on
earth, and no two have exactly the same face, the same features,
the same handwriting, the same personality. Even twins are
different; they are not exactly alike. Why? Because the Creator
wants it that way. He is a great lover of variety, diversity, and
individuality.

Life has endowed us with the basis for a personality, plus the privilege and the responsibility of unfolding, developing, and perfecting it with distinct, individual characteristics. Your personality will be singular in this world; it is guaranteed that it will duplicate no other one. Is it not a stupendous task to enfold and perfect such an individual personality? And this responsibility is yours and mine. There is no chance of distributing it to anyone else, nor can we dispense with it. It is the very purpose of life, the very reason why we are here. There is no escape from the problem; we just have to solve it.

One day, we will meet the Lifegiver, the great I AM, and then and there we will have to render account of what we have done with that precious talent—that person—He committed into our care. Have we developed and perfected a personality in His likeness? There is only one thing we can do: develop, cultivate, and perfect our personality (this course is designed to help attain this aim), or carelessly neglect this responsibility, forfeit our opportunity, and retard and even mutilate our personality. If you choose the first, the result will be eternal bliss; if you choose the second, it will be eternal destruction. The former choice is the only life worth living, isn't it? Therefore always give preference to the development and perfection of your personality.

You have the green light to win a place side by side with the highest and noblest personalities this world has brought forth. Your future and destiny are in your hands. This is one of the basic principles of Christianity. Whether white or colored, master or servant, you, and you alone, control your future and your destiny. You are not a tumbleweed to be blown hither and yon by every gust of wind. The power to be what you want to be, to get what you desire, and to accomplish whatever you strive for is promised you and abides within your reach. It rests solely with you whether you step forward to develop and perfect your personality to the highest degree possible. If you want to improve the world, the first step is to improve yourself. Develop enthusiasm, ambition, strengthen your will power, and you will make your personality what it should be. Remember the

wise saying: "Many an ill can be cured by just prefixing it with a
w." And Oliver Townsend says:

> Let me be upright, stable, strong,
> As the linden tree, that stood so long
> In my garden.

Great nations and great communities are made up of great personalities. They are distinguished by superior qualities, especially
of mind and heart. These personalities have great vision, lofty
ideals, unselfish motives, moral courage, stout hearts,
self-control, unquenchable faith, practical wisdom, and sterling
characters. There is no valid reason why you cannot learn from
these torch-bearers who have gone before us. Follow them; be one
of them.

THE   FIRST   IMPRESSION

The impression we first make upon the world is a physical one.
Before a word is spoken, long before any intellectual or spiritual
qualities are disclosed, it is the physical part of our personality
that is either impressive or insignificant to others. Therefore, in
our study, because of this obvious and practical reason, we shall
reverse St. Paul's arrangement. He enumerates the parts of our
personality—spirit, soul, and body—by starting with the spiritual
and closing with the body, the physical, whereas we shall start
with the body, the physical, and close with the spiritual.

The first impression you give of your physical personality as a
whole is of the utmost importance. Is your body weak, frail, and
sickly; or strong, hale, and healthy? Tall or small, fat or slender,
bent or upright? The physical personality conveys vastly more to
the world than just our frame, image, color, and form. Our
countenance registers the fact of youth or age, male or female,
intelligence or stupidity, joy and happiness or pain and misery. It
also expresses attributes of the human soul and spirit-friendliness
or enmity, hope or despair, optimism or pessimism, trust or doubt,
faith or unbelief, agreement or opposition, peace

or discord. Thus one experienced in human relations can read and interpret a great deal about a person he meets by the impression that the physical personality makes at the first meeting. Of course, to be able to pass a correct judgment, one should not be influenced by emotions, or likes and dislikes, or the judgment will be biased, colored, and will lose its intellectual value. After you have been introduced to a person you usually say: "I am very glad to meet you." But seldom do you feel what you say. It is just conventionality. When you really feel glad to meet a person you will show it and express it, and your new acquaintance will feel that you are a fine personality. What arouses appreciation and emotion in a first impression is a vital part of one's personality. It is a reflection of the inward self. Or, as Oliver Wendell Holmes puts it:

> The outward forms the inward man reveal—
> We guess the pulp before we cut the peel.

SOME RULES FOR EVERY DAY

Subject yourself daily to a severe self-examination. Ask yourself and answer the following questions:

1. What kind of an impression does my personality make on others?

2. Is my *physical* personality (my body) in buoyant, vibrant health and natural beauty?

3. Is my *intellectual* personality (my character, or soul) praiseworthy, an exemplification and a likeness of Christ?

4. Do I have a pleasant and forceful *spiritual* personality with which to glorify my Father in heaven?

5. What am I doing to perfect my personality?

6. What efforts do I put forth to overcome faulty habits?

Emily May Young, says:

> Earthly desires keep men in bondage;
> Only the overcomer is free.
> They are the souls attaining perfection,
> Changing from anguish to felicity.

4. THE BODY

AMONG ALL the forms of life we perceive on earth, man is the masterpiece; he is life supreme. Therefore the first and indispensable requisite for a charming, vigorous personality is vibrant, vigorous health and vitality. Perfection cannot be attained with a diseased body. That is the logical reason why, in our personality-building program, we must start by building a healthful body. Without it we can do very little. Health, vigor, vitality—these are the things so seriously needed today. The National Research Council presents us with these startling findings: 97,000,000 Americans are chronically ill with one kind of ailment or another. Ten million children have bad teeth; six million people suffer from glandular disturbances, four million are undernourished, one million have tuberculosis, and one million have spinal curvatures. Is this not a most pitiful picture of the most prosperous nation on earth? What must we do?

With the first dawn of reason, the human mind should begin to regard intelligently the physical structure of the human body. Here, Jehovah has given a specimen of himself, for man was made in the image of God.

God himself made the human body. It is the most exquisite, most wonderful organism that has come to us from the Divine hand. King David esteemingly commands:

. . . thou hast covered me in my mother's womb.
I will praise thee; for I am fearfully and wonderfully made: . . .
Thine eyes did see my substance, yet being unperfect; and in thy book all my members were written, which in continuance were fashioned, when as yet there was none of them. (Ps. 139: 13,14,16.)

The supreme importance of the body is shown by the fact that God, the architect, drew a plan that contained the various parts of the body—bones, muscles, nerves, blood vessels, tissues, and organs. The Book that contains this plan is another of those wonderful volumes to be found in God's library. "We shall be studying these books throughout eternity," says Dr. A. I. Brown in God and You. And he continues: "The great care exercised in the creation of the body can be understood when we remember I Corinthians 3:16,17: 'Know ye not that ye are the temple of God, and that the Spirit of God dwelleth in you? . . . The temple of God is holy, which temple ye are.'"

The truth enunciated here is beyond our comprehension. But in some mysterious way it tells us that the Third Person of the Trinity has taken up His residence within us. How this is accomplished is impossible to understand, but the sublimity of the idea ought to lead us to a profound care of our body, since we have such a guest.

E. G. White says: "When human agents choose to do the will of God, and conform to the character of Christ, our Creator and Savior, He will act through their bodily organs and faculties." How wonderful! Can we comprehend this?

"Can any honor exceed that which has been conferred on the human body? . . . Can any power exceed its power? Can any glory exceed the glory with which he is invested? No wonder that the Apostle Paul beseeches men to present their bodies as a living sacrifice to God," remarks Dr. Pulsford.

Yes, God requires all men to render their bodies to Him a living sacrifice, not a dead or dying sacrifice, with their own various courses of action debilitating them and filling them with impurities and disease. How often, against better counsel, one hears: "That's my own business. It's my body. I can do with it as I please—smoke, drink, or anything else." No less a man than the great philosopher and Apostle Paul gives us the answer to that: "What! know ye that ... ye are not your own? For ye are bought with a price: therefore glorify God in your body, and in your spirit, which are God's." (I Cor. 6:19-20.)

Indeed, we are not our own. Our body has been purchased with a great price, even the suffering and death of the Son of

God. If we would understand this, and fully realize it, we would feel a great responsibility resting upon us to keep our body in the best condition of health. But when we take courses that expend our vitality, decrease our strength, and becloud our intellect, we sin against our Creator; we do not glorify him in our body and spirit, says E. G. White.

Is it not our duty to *know how* to preserve our body in the very best condition of health? And is it not a sacred obligation to live up to the light that God graciously is giving us? If we close our eyes to the light for fear we shall see our wrongs, which we are unwilling to forsake, shall such a course not multiply our guilt and convince us of our wickedness? Is it possible to love God with all our heart, mind, soul, and strength, while we are loving appetite and taste a great deal more? Of course not! Would it not seem that what we love more than our Lord becomes our idol, and thus would we not become idol worshipers, transgressors of the moral code? Therefore, let us not through wrong habits lessen our strength, or lose our hold on life, and forfeit the perfection of our personality. Devitalizing habits of eating, drinking, and living sometimes seem to give temporary solace and pleasure, but they slowly poison the body and deaden the nerves.

Make it your purpose positively to cultivate a love for life-life here and life eternal. That's the best, most effective opponent of all harmful, health-destroying habits. Make perfection of living your hobby. Thus you will not only keep free from weakness and illness, but develop health and charm to their utmost degree. And if you are of the female gender, you will find no need to impress the masters of creation with superficial pretense. All your loveliness and charm will be natural. When the Creator made lovely Eve—and she must have been beautiful-it was her loveliness that forced upon Adam the decision not to stay in Paradise alone, but to follow Eve into exile. And all her loveliness and beauty was real and natural. God gave no make-up kit to Eve with which to counterfeit beauty.

God made provision to overcome *all* bad habits. Perfect

health of body, mind, and spirit is within reach of everyone, who desires strongly enough to acquaint himself with Nature's laws and restorative methods, and who is willing to do the simple things necessary to bring into existence *perfect health and vitality.*

Health affects your personality. It is of paramount importance in personality engineering. Not only in your physical part, but also in your mental and spiritual parts, though all manifestations of personality have their roots in the physical part, the body. Abnormal social behavior, evil-doing, criminality, and sin of every description are the result of physical degeneration. The Savior of the world looked at, and treated, sinners as afflicted, ailing, sick, and injured victims, who were greatly in need of a physician and of treatment. Preserving health is therefore a moral and religious duty, for health is the basis of all social, mental, and spiritual virtues. We can be no longer useful when we are not well.

Health is a great treasure, the richest blessing mortals can possess. Anything and everything, wealth and honor, riches and learning, are dearly purchased if they are bought at the loss of vigor and vitality, strength and health.

Health is an achievement of which few appreciate the great value, yet upon it the efficiency of your physical, mental, and spiritual power largely depends. Our body is the habitation of our soul, intellect, mind, and emotions.

In building your personality, you are duty bound to become acquainted with and receive an intelligent knowledge of the wonderful human body, its physical structure, the laws of life, and the health principles that control it. He who remains in willing ignorance about his physical being, and violates the laws of health through ignorance, is sinning against God our Creator, in whose image we are made. The physical body must have special care, so that the indwelling powers may not be dwarfed, but can develop to their fullest extent and capacity. The person who does not control health is neglecting the very first principle in personality engineering.

I am building a body for Jesus,
    To be of some service for Him;
I pray that He'll help me remember
    My purpose, which must not grow dim.

He says that it is His temple,
    Kept holy and clean it must be.
He left us this word in the Bible;
    I'm sure it was written for me.

So daily in true consideration
    I bow at His feet, and I pray
That I may but realize His watchcare
    O'er all my members each day.

For what is more wonderful truly
    Than physical laws God has made?
Each fiber and nerve of my being
    Has on it these principles laid.

Whether I'm eating or drinking,
    Or working or resting, 'twere well
To do everything to God's glory
    And all selfish motives repel.

Not only for this day I'm building,
    But for days that shall lengthen to years,
When the harvest of souls shall be ended
    And the sign of the Saviour appears.

                             AUTHOR UNKNOWN

5. THE AMAZING PROTOPLASM

IT IS common knowledge that all living matter originates in a tiny little cell of protoplasm one twenty-fifth of an inch in diameter. The human body is made up of at least twenty-six trillion protoplasmic cells. Each tiny cell consists of about 72 per cent oxygen, 13 1/2 per cent carbon, 9 per cent hydrogen, 2 1/2 per cent nitrogen, and small amounts of the following twelve elements: calcium, sodium, chlorine, fluorine, manganese, phosphorus, sulphur, potassium, magnesium, iron, silicon, and iodine. The human body—its bones, flesh, blood, brain, nerves, skin, hair, and nails—is entirely made of these tiny protoplasmic cells. They are the most mysterious things that can engage the investigatory talent of the human mind. Protoplasm is *living matter*. It is irritable (not wanting to be touched). It is active (metabolism), it builds the food we eat into higher forms (anabolism), and it breaks down used up and useless cells (catabolism). Dr. A. I. Brown declares:

Let your imagination have full rein now as you attempt to picture what is happening inside of these miraculous little blobs of protoplasmic jelly. Wonder of wonders! The central portion, or nucleus, with its 48 chromosomes, now undergoes a process of multiplication and instead of 48 there are 96. Half of these rush to one end of the jelly-ball and half to the other end, awaiting the next step, which occurs immediately. This is done in such a way that each new cell finds itself possessed of exactly 48 chromosomes.

The male and female cells, known respectively as the sperm and the ovum, contain, of course, these bits of chromatin. The essential contents of these nuclear elements are called chromosomes, which may be described as strings of beads, the latter bearing the name of genes carry in their tiny bodies all the characteristics of the human body. For instance, one bead has the hair color, another the shape of the nose, others the shape of the mouth, contour of the face, and so on. You are what you are, then, because of your chromosomes. The progeny of that first tiny cell, number, in every human body, at least twenty-six thousand billion. What an astonishing family! We may think, then, of our bodies as huge cities, the inhabitants of which are these billions of little "people," all specialists of one kind or another.

There are carpenters, masons, plasterers and plumbers; electricians, ordinary laborers, scavengers, gardeners, and cooks; servants, policemen, soldiers, sailors, lawyers, merchants and doctors. Here is a busy, peaceful, harmonious city, the citizens of which carry on ceaselessly, night and day, immense and complex industries. They work independently and yet very dependently. If one group, for any reason, were to stop work, all other groups would die. Every part must be kept in health in order that the welfare of the whole may be preserved.

One may ask: How long can these tiny protoplasm workers live and work? Here is an answer:

Dr. Woodruff kept a one-cell paramecium growing to more than 10,000 generations, and the original parent was still alive and going strong. With this fact in mind, if a protoplasmic cell could live to the age of a human, proportionately its life span would be 250,000 years.

Dr. A. I. Brown asks: "Would Adam and Eve have lived forever, if sin had not taken possession?" It is something to think about.

Materialists do not want to believe in God the Creator. But no scientist, dead or alive, has been able to solve the mystery of protoplasm without Him. When we consider the life principle in protoplasm, we are in the presence of "the great I AM."

Protoplasm is "protein," and the human body is made and kept in good condition by protein. That is why doctors and nutritionists always stress the importance of protein foods, of a sufficient amount, and intake, as well as the right combination.

Protoplasm is *living matter*; it acts, it eats, it must be fed, and if it is not fed right it gets sick, and dies. All sickness has its origin right here. It's a matter of eating the right food, the right amount, and the right combination. Failure to do this will unfailingly show up in deficiency, in ailments, and in the indisposition of body and mind. Thus we can understand the saying of the Greek sage, Hippocrates: "Let food be your medicine and medicine be your food."

In our personality engineering, "eat to live, eat intelligently and scientifically" is of paramount importance.

6. THE FUNCTIONS OF THE FOOD SUPPLY

Man's rich with little were his judgment true;
Nature is frugal and her wants are few.
These few wants answered, bring sincere delights;
But fools create themselves new appetites.

EDWARD YOUNG

Gluttony is the source of all our infirmities, and the fountain of all our diseases. As an oil lamp is chocked by a super abundance of oil, and a fire extinguished by excess of fuel, so is the natural heat of the body by intemperate diet.

ROBERT BURTON

HUNGER is man's greatest friend, but appetite his basest enemy. Taste and hunger will select man's food supply on a scientific basis. But ignorance, abuse, and willful neglect have debased and depraved appetite until it has become man's deepest curse. Man's appetite for strong drink has wrecked many a fortune, existence, home, family, and life's happiness. Man's appetite dethrones his reason, destroys his will, dulls his intellect, and ruins his soul.

Man's depraved appetite for the wrong kind of food is almost as pernicious as his appetite for strong drink. The curse of a depraved appetite for the wrong food is that it gnaws at man's vitals until it destroys the grace and beauty of his form, and with it his physical personality.

Indiscriminate eating and overeating are called the crimes of the American people against their own bodies, which, as a result, fill hospitals and graves. Scientists and physicians declare that the alarming increase in the death rate from heart, liver, and kidney diseases is caused by overeating and improper, unscientific diet.

The digestive organs can digest only a certain amount of food; all surplus food must be digested bacterially in the stomach, duodenum, and intestines. This means that all foods that are not digested by the digestive fluids must decompose, putrefy, and decay in the digestive organs. This causes the generation of poisonous gases that can be neither digested nor assimilated, but are carried by the lymph and blood stream through the whole system. This can induce what is called autointoxication, which is the foundation for a multitude of diseases.

Years ago, when doing some postgraduate work, I attended a small but highly efficient school of the drugless healing art, the Sierra State University, in Los Angeles. One day, when studying sinusitis, the professor, Dr. Flodin, was asked: "What is the best approach to correct this disorder?" "Cleanse the colon" came the prompt answer, with the following explanation: "The poisons from the intestines generate through the whole body, accumulate and settle at the weakest points in the system. In our case it is the sinus. The principle is, go after the cause and the effect will take care of itself." It made sense and the lesson stuck.

Thus we see that the success of our building program depends largely on our eating habits. No matter what you eat, or how much you eat, your food counts either for you or against you. The food you eat can be either wholesome or poisonous to your system, can form you or deform you, can make you attractive or unattractive, can make you beautiful or graceless.

Even the most wholesome food, if eaten in abnormal amounts or in incorrect combinations, can become a poison to your system and a liability to your personality. For example: the wrong selection or an excessive intake of food may cause a torpid liver. A torpid liver can produce a morbid mind, and it is a morbid mind that creates immoral thoughts and leads to base actions. Likewise a sour, dyspeptic stomach can result in an acid temper, and an overloaded or sluggish liver can cause a choleric, angry disposition.

Man's nature—intellectual, moral, and spiritual—is so dependent on the condition of his physical being that food almost seems the prime element to consider, and its study a real science in human life. It is through food that the body is built and maintained. Scientifically, food is divided into three classes, protein, carbohydrates, and fats, according to their function.

PROTEIN

What is protein and what is its function? The meaning of the word gives it its proper standing among the classes of food. The word means "of prime importance" and that is exactly what protein is in our physical economy—of prime importance, nothing more and nothing less. It is protein that gives people a pleasing, shapely form; it gives the countenance its beauty, the eyes their sparkle, the hair a natural radiance, and the skin an enticing, velvety texture. It is protein that makes the muscles firm and the nerves steady.

Every cell in the body (there are more than 26 trillion of them) is constructed of protoplasma, which is protein. Protein is the essential material for body building and the building of tissue, and we also need it for the maintenance of health and happiness.

Without protein all else is of no avail. Carbohydrates, fats, minerals, vitamins—all are useless without protein. It must be available in sufficient quantities, or the body cannot build and repair, generate and regenerate, the cells that form the tissues of the body. Every cell in our body is constructed and composed of protoplasma, and protoplasma is protein, the end product of all our nutrition.

What then is this mysterious substance, protein? It is a composition of amino acids (synonym: food acids) in various forms. And amino acids are chemical compounds composed of the following "atoms": nitrogen, hydrogen, oxygen, and carbon. In addition, some have atoms of sulphur, iodine, iron, phosphorus, and other elements. Protein compounds are the most complex of all chemical compounds; they contain thousands of atoms in each molecule. The amino acids form the blood plasma, the building material of all the cells in the human system. Therefore the amino acids are known as the building blocks of the human body.

These amino acids are the only nitrogenous compounds in the human economy. In our study we have found that nitrogen is the marvelous element that protects us from the greatest disaster that could befall us, namely, to be burned up by oxygen. If the material known as protein lacked the nitrogen element, we would be burned up like everything else we eat and drink, classed as carbohydrates and fats. These are mercilessly burned up in our body, and what is left is ash, because these compounds of carbohydrates and fats lack the protective element, nitrogen.

We all know that ash is useless as a building material. So we can easily comprehend that there is no building-material value in carbohydrates and fats.

The only and best source of a complete protein is in all vegetables and fruits. In short, it is found in plant life. I said, the *only* and the *best*, and I mean just that. This is contrary to the common belief that perfect protein is found in meat and flesh food. But that belief is erroneous. Science conclusively has proved that there is no perfect protein aside from that found in the vegetable kingdom.

All the atoms of which protein (the amino acids) is compounded are found abundantly in all plant life, vegetables, and fruits. All these atoms of the vegetable kingdom are organic, which means they are "alive" with vitality.

The mineral kingdom contains all the atoms of which this world is made, but in an inorganic (death) form, that is, "lifeless atoma." We know that we cannot eat stones or sand, any inorganic mineral, in short, and stay alive. The mineral kingdom lacks the life principle. (We will study in another chapter the wonderful story of the mysteries of the life principle.) Here it will suffice to say that the Creator sent life into the atoms of vegetation by means of sun rays. And in this way, and in this way only, lifeless atoms are changed into life atoms, or vital atoms. This is the change from inorganic to organic matter, whereas death is the change from organic back into inorganic matter. There is no other way known to the science of biology whereby lifeless atoms can be changed into life atoms, save by way of the vegetable kingdom. Therefore we cannot live without plants, vegetables, grain, nuts, and fruits. This also is the logical reason why the Creator first called into being the vegetable kingdom, and only afterward the animal kingdom and man. It is in the vegetable kingdom that we find the fascinating story of protein.

The atoms of meat and flesh food are vital as long as the animal is alive, but within six minutes after being slaughtered, all life in the atoms desists and ceases. Therefore flesh protein consists of "lifeless, dead, inorganic atoms." Scientifically, and by right, meat protein cannot be called a perfect protein, because it does not contain all the amino acids, and the important life principle is missing. It remains a fact that dead protein is secondhand protein, and an emergency measure only. God allowed it after the deluge, when the entire vegetable kingdom was destroyed, and no perfect protein was available.

Vitality, life, is vibration, and science declares that the vibration of the protoplasma, which is protein, stops within minutes after death occurs.

Judge for yourself. Can such a type of protein justly be called a perfect and complete protein? You say no, and you are right. The main factor for a complete protein—the life factor—is missing. And this life principle can be found only, but abundantly, in the vegetable kingdom. Dead atoms, as found in the meat of dead animals, are doomed to putrefaction and disintegration. But to build a personality full of life, of vim and vigor, we need life atoms full of vitality. Science declares: "Life only begets life."

When the amino-acid foods are of live organic origin, they perform on the highest level of organic efficiency. Life then becomes dynamic, organic, fluent, vibrant, impregnated with vitality. But those amino acids that are the constitutive elements of the protein in the food we eat can only be obtained by us through the proper intake of a variety of foods rich in protein.

These proteins, however, must be alive with the ingredients of life, the life force itself, in order to have the life-giving, life-generating power required for proper cell, blood, muscle, gland, and organ regeneration and repair. This means that we must seek and obtain our protein from plant life food. As stated before, all vegetables and fruits contain these necessary elements, but the queen of protein foods is the soybean. The soybean contains twenty of the twenty-three amino acids, which is probably the highest protein and biological value known in the vegetable kingdom.

For the new-born baby, provision has been made in milk. The nitrogenous (protein) part of the mother's milk contains eighteen of the twenty-three amino acids; it is a complete and adequate protein. The protein of the milk is quite readily and easily digested by the enzyme rennin, missing in adults; therefore milk is not the best source of protein for adults.

Protein from the slaughtered bodies of animals has no life-giving, regenerating power, as we have said. Life and vitality is lost immediately upon the killing of an animal, and the vital factors involved in the function of the amino-acid combination are lost.

Vegetables, fruits, nuts, and grains are Nature's storehouses of protein. They contain all the necessary atomic constituents from which our body can form amino acids of the finest life-giving kind. In the consumption of meat and flesh products, we stress again, there is no life, only excessive accumulations of all sorts detrimental to life, including a high percentage of uric acid.

Dr. W. L. Abt, in *The Key*, concludes:

> Plants, vegetables, fruits and nuts, are nature's vital store houses of proteins and other vital ingredients for the promotion of life. They contain the proteins which the body requires for rebuilding worn out and damaged cells and tissues, and the amino acids building bricks, or atomic constituents of these proteins; and they contain them in vital, living, fresh and uncontaminated purity, in a form which is obtainable nowhere else in the whole world.

There is no substitute for the life of fruits, plants, nuts, and their amino-acid constituents. The first health teacher of man, the Creator himself, planted a garden eastward in Eden, pleasant to the sight, and good for food. (Gen. 1:29; 2:8.)

> God Almighty first planted a garden
> And indeed it is the purest of human pleasures.
> In the kiss of the sun there is pardon,
> In the song of a bird there is mirth;
> We are nearer God's heart in a garden
> Than anywhere else on the earth.
>
> FRANCIS BACON

CARBOHYDRATES, FATS AND THEIR FUNCTIONS

Carbohydrates are the starch and sugar foods we consume. Fats are the oils and all fatty substances in the foods. Both carbohydrates and fats are chemical compounds of carbon, hydrogen, and oxygen. These compounds are important in the life process, but of no use as material for body building.

When we feed an engine gasoline and oil, the chemical change (combustion) results in heat and energy. When we feed the body carbohydrates and fat, the chemical change (metabolism) results in heat and energy.

An engine of considerable weight may need only a small amount of gasoline and oil to run for one day and do a day's work. The human economy likewise needs but a comparatively small amount of carbohydrates for heat and energy. Older textbooks claimed that quite a large percentage of carbohydrates was needed for energy fuel, but recent medical research has proved this claim erroneous; a very moderate use of carbohydrates and a liberal use of fat are now recommended by medical authorities for human heat and energy.

Of the different kinds of fats, we shall consider for our study two classes: the saturated and the unsaturated fats. These are chemical terms that differentiate between the molecular combinations that make up the two fats. In general, saturated fats are triglyceride animal fats. Unsaturated (polyunsaturated) fats are vegetable fats of linoleic acid, which is unsaturated fatty acid. (Some fish oils also contain unsaturated fatty acids.) Safflower oil contains the highest percentage—75 per cent.

Remember this: Unsaturated fatty acid is not found in meat or dairy products. Unsaturated (polyunsaturated) fats decrease the cholesterol level in the body. Saturated (animal) fats raise the cholesterol level.

Unsaturated fats preserve the protein in the body. Carbohydrates rob the body of protein. Therefore it seems only common sense to follow medical advice, and for body heat and energy use carbohydrates sparingly and unsaturated fats liberally.

It has been proved that the human body has an unlimited capacity to burn up fats, but only a very limited amount of carbohydrates.

The foregoing, in short, is the story of carbohydrates, fats, and their functions. For regenerative work, and to keep the body in good shape, youthful and beautiful, we need a large amount of protein, about 30 per cent of our food intake.

You probably have heard doctors say of some people that they are overfed but undernourished. These people eat an excessive amount of starches, fats, and sweets, but not enough of the wonderful protein foods from the Garden of Eden. If you belong to this class, take heed!

Here is what Dr. Victor H. Lindlar says:

> The truth is, you cannot build blood out of fat, starch or sugar. If that could be done, we would not see so many stout people suffering from anemia. They have not eaten enough of the food necessary to make good red blood, but they have eaten too much of the food easily turned into unneeded, unhealthy fat.
>
> Actually, body food, like a lot of coal, has only one real purpose, to serve as a source of stored energy and heat. Coal has its place in your house, and in a locomotive, where it supplies the energy that turns the wheels. But you don't use coal to

build the walls of a house, railroads don't use coal to construct a locomotive, and neither can you use fat to build the human body.

What are the specific foods you should have on your diet list? Fruits like: apricots, peaches, pears, apples, pineapple, prunes, raisins, strawberries, etc. Vegetables like: lettuce, cucumbers, watercress, spinach, carrots, parsley, etc. These are items to star on your menu if you need to build up the life-giving fluid which courses through your body.

It is no problem to build good red blood and at the same time avoid surplus calories, but it is difficult to build good red blood when you are eating too many starches, sweets and fats.

This statement comes from E. G. White:

> God has given us an ample variety of healthful foods, and each person should choose from it the things that experience and sound judgment prove to be best suited to his own necessities. Nuts and nut foods are coming largely into use to take the place of flesh meats. With nuts may be combined grains, fruits, and some roots, to make foods that are healthful and nourishing.

The great amount of water in meat is not "clean" water, but water saturated with uric acid and other residues.

To those who assert that meat is a superior food and a complete protein, I recommend the study of the above chart. If there still should be any doubt, let us prove the truth.

Take any kind of nut or bean and at the right time put it in the ground. What will happen? Within a few weeks a little plant will peep above the surface. Now haul the dead cow into the stable and see if she will bear a calf. If the flesh still had "life atoms," like the nut or the bean, should not the same thing happen? We know it will not, because of the truth we have stated.

In the vegetable organism the constructive life force is at work, combining inorganic material into complex organic compounds, in either a tree, plant, or, in the human body, blood plasma and tissue—life tissue.

In the dead animal organism the destructive death forces are

simultaneously active in the process of disintegration and putrefaction. Meat is dead protein, of all foods the most toxic. It is a
waste product and poisonous to the human body, if not eliminated
quickly.

The following table* gives the average composition of nuts
and meat. And remember that the atoms in nuts are vital-alive,
whereas in meat they are *stagnant-dead.*

AVERAGE CHEMICAL COMPOSITION OF PROTEIN FOODS

Water	Protein		Fat	Carbo-hydrates	Mineral matter
Complete protein: life atoms.					
Organic unsaturated fat.					
Almond	4.9	21.4	54.4	16.8	2.5
Almond butter	2.2	21.7	61.5	11.6	3.0
Brazilnut	4.7	17.4	65.0	9.6	3.3
Butternut	4.5	27.9	61.2	3.4	3.0
Coconut	13.0	6.6	56.2	22.6	1.6
Chestnut	6.1	10.7	7.8	73.0	2.4
Peanut	7.4	29.8	43.5	17.1	2.2
Peanut butter	2.1	29.3	46.5	17.1	5.0
Pecan	3.4	12.1	70.7	12.2	1.6
Pignolia	6.2	33.9	48.2	7.9	3.8
Walnut (black)	2.5	27.6	56.3	11.7	1.9
Walnut (English)	2.5	18.4	64.4	13.0	1.7
Beans (dried)	12.6	22.5	1.8	59.6	3.5
Soya beans	10.0	35.0	2.1	30.0	3.5
Incomplete protein: death.					
Inorganic toxic fat (cholesterol).					
Meat (average)	72.0	20.0	5.0	.4	1.1
Beef	76.0	18.0	5.0	..	1.0
Chicken	72.2	21.3	4.5	.7	.9
Clam	85.8	8.6	1.0	2.0	2.6
Fish (average	80.0	18.0	.8	..	1.2
Lobster	79.2	16.4	1.8	.4	2.2
Oyster	86.9	6.2	1.2	3.7	1.4
Pork	75.0	20.25	6.8	..	.7

* This analysis and comparison is taken from *Vital Facts About Foods,* by
Otto Carque.

7. PERSONALITY ENGINEERING

BUILDING THE PHYSICAL
PERSONALITY

WHEN GOD created the world, he made a variety of chemical elements. Science has discovered 102 of them, to date. When I went to school, nearly fifty years ago, we knew only 92. How many elements science will have discovered by the year 2000, if time lasts, nobody knows. Sixteen of these elements are the material our physical body is made of, and science assures us positively that these sixteen elements in our physical entity are exactly the same as those found in the ground. Science verifies therewith the report of the creation in the Holy Scripture, which declares: "God the Eternal molded man from the dust of the ground" (Gen. 2:7).

Thus both Revelation and science give an unmistakable direction in which to look for the material to build and replenish our physical body. Look to the ground—to the soil, from which you are made.

A very good introduction to this subject can be found in the little volume Are You What You Eat, by H. E. Kirschner, M.D., and Herbert C. White, A.B.* Dr. J. C. Walter, who wrote the introduction, states:

To the question: "What is going on in the living soil?" Dr. Kirschner and Mr. White explain very thoroughly the characteristics of the soil, and reiterate the research findings of many scientists that good, fertile soil, free of chemical sprays, provides essential nutrients for plants and animals. These nutrients offer superior food elements which are basic for optimum health.

---

* Published by H. C. White Publications, P.O. Box 8014, La Sierra, California.

And in the preface the authors say:

> Our bodies are built from the food we eat. There is a constant breaking down of the tissues of the body; every movement of every organ involves waste, and this waste is repaired from our food. Each organ of the body requires its share of nutrition. The brain must be supplied with its portion; the bones, muscles, and nerves demand theirs. It is a wonderful process that transforms the food into blood, and *uses this blood to build up the varied parts of the body.*

The Creator planned his creatures to have proper food to live. In order to know what the best foods are, we must study God's original plan for man's diet.

In Moffatt's translation of the Bible the report of the Creation reads as follows: "So God formed man in His own likeness, and said: 'See, I give you *every plant* that bears seed all over the earth—and every tree with seed in its fruits; *be that your food*'" (Gen. 1:29).

Accordingly, He placed on earth a great variety of nutritious substances, in a manner delightful to the eye, palatable to the taste, and easily accessible to men. Thus: "In the land of Eden, to the far east, God the Eternal then planted a park, where he put the man whom He had molded. And from *the ground* God the Eternal made all sorts of trees to grow that were delightful to see and *good to eat*" (Gen. 2:8-9).

Here is the diet the Creator chose and prepared for us to build and maintain our earthly temple: all seed-bearing plants and all seed-bearing fruits, commonly known as vegetables, grains (seed-bearing plants), and fruits (seed-bearing fruits). This provision evidently embraced the finer vegetable growth, since every green herb was designated as food for the beasts.

In this divine menu for man we do not find the main course of the bill of fare of people today, that is, steak, chops, roasts, and all the other common flesh foods from dead animals. Since the habit of eating the flesh, fat, and even the blood of animal corpses is the custom of today, and since it is commonly believed that this food is a necessity to build and maintain the human-body economy, we shall investigate this type of material and the custom in a special chapter.

Primarily, we must have a sufficient knowledge of the material we are made of, if we are to choose intelligently the type of food necessary for building material, for the maintenance of our physical entity. Therefore let us solve the following questions:

What is the analysis of the human body?

What are the names of the 16 elements we are made of?

What is the proportion of each element?

Where can they be obtained?

One writer humorously gives the following analysis of a person weighing about 150 pounds:

Enough water to fill a 10 gallon keg.

Enough fat to make seven bars of soap.

Enough carbon to make 9,000 lead pencils.

Enough iron to make a medium nail.

Enough phosphorus to make 2,200 match tips.

Enough potassium to explode a toy cannon.

Enough sugar to fill a table sugar shaker.

Enough calcium to whitewash a chicken coop.

Enough sulfur to treat a dog and rid him of fleas.

Enough magnesium to make one dose of salts.

Enough iodine to make one drop of tincture of iodine.

And as much oxygen as there is in 15,000 quarts of air.

And the whole supply would be worth on the common market about 98 cents. We can be happy that the value of a personality is not measured in these terms and in mathematical figures. But here are figures in pounds and ounces:

Oxygen	88	lbs.	Sulphur	3 1/4	oz.
Carbon	37	"	Sodium	3 1/2	"
Hydrogen	14	"	Fluorine	2 1/2	"
Nitrogen	3 1/2	"	Magnesium	2 1/2	"
Calcium	3 1/2	"	Iron	1 3/4	"
Phosphorus	3 1/4	"	Silicon	1 1/4	"
Chlorine	1/2	"	Manganese	1/2	"
Potassium	1/4	"	Iodine	1/4	"

The first six elements—oxygen, carbon, hydrogen, nitrogen, calcium, and phosphorus—make up 99 per cent of the body and the remaining one per cent is made up of the other ten afore-mentioned mineral elements in small quantities, and they are just as important as the major ones. These chemical elements, found in the air and in the soil, are used by nature to build the various cells of which the different tissues and organs are made. Each type of cell has to be built with its own particular chemical, if it is to function normally and well. Now let us study these different chemical elements and find out where they are to be found.

1. *Oxygen* is the most important chemical in the human body. About 67 per cent of our body is oxygen. Any deficiency of it will lead to serious consequences. Supply the needs by (a) breathing fresh air deeply, and (b) drinking raw fruit and vegetable juices freely. They abundantly supply organic oxygen.

2. *Carbon* is fatty food. We need only one third as much as oxygen. An oversupply will be destructive. It lubricates and heats the body. The need should be supplied by nuts, nut butter, almonds (very good), avocados, sweet potatoes, and olives.

3. *Hydrogen* keeps the body cool and youthful. It is the medium through which all the material in the body is trans ported, in or out. It also is a preventive against inflammation. Supply the need from all watery vegetables and fruits such as lettuce, cucumbers, carrots, parsnips, celery, tomatoes, peaches, pears, berry, fruit, and vegetable juices of all kinds, and water. It is one of the chief elements in the composition and maintenance of physical life, and fills a decisive role in forming compounds essential to life.

4. *Nitrogen* dilutes the oxygen in the system and prevents it from burning up the body. If this stabilizer gets below normal, oxygen becomes a destroyer. Nitrogen keeps the body tissue in a balanced, fresh condition. Supply the need for nitrogen from foods rich in nitrogen, such as beans, soybeans, mung beans, peas, lentils, soy milk, whole wheat, rye, millet, all kinds of raw nuts, and alfalfa.

5. *Calcium* builds teeth and bones, gives strength and firm-

ness to the arteries, increases the life of the cells, and aids in the assimilation of several of the other elements. It is found in (fruits) lemons, pineapples, limes, grapefruit, oranges, unsulfured dried fruits, apples, all berries, and all nuts except peanuts; (vegetables) spinach, broccoli, cauliflower, asparagus, turnips, okra, parsnips, all green leafy vegetables, onions, garlic, and potatoes; and in milk.

6. *Sodium* is essential for the production of the electrical induction current that is generated in the brain and the spinal cord. Sodium is a body cleanser, and of vital importance to the blood and glands. It should be received from organic sources. This means through plant life, rather than from inorganic sources like white table salt, which should be used moderately. It is an aid in the digestion of albumin, protein, and fats, and keeps a certain amount of calcium and magnesium in a liquid state. Supply the need from (fruits) peaches, figs, apples, unsulfured dried fruits, berries of all kinds, grapes, dates, and raw nuts, and (vegetables) celery, carrots, cucumbers, radishes, squash, beets, also the leaves of beets, dandelion greens, and leeks.

7. *Chlorine* is, with sodium, a cleanser, and unites in the body with other elements to form salts that are indispensable for good health and a vibrant body. Supply the need from (vegetables) lettuce, cabbage, cucumbers, raw carrots, radishes, eggplant, parsnips, asparagus, beets, sweet potatoes, avocados, tomatoes, coconuts, and pomegranates; (grains) whole wheat, rye, millet, and brown rice; and from salt.

8. *Fluorine* acts as a cement; it knits the bones together, aids in making the enamel of the teeth, strengthens the tendons, and helps in the formation of the blood cells. It must be taken from organic sources. Its inorganic form is a poison, used to kill rats. Regrettably, it is also used in water enforcement. Only fluorine from the vegetable kingdom is suitable for utilization by the human body. Supply the need from vegetables rich in fluorine such as onions, garlic, beets, all greens, raw cabbage, lettuce, watercress, green peas, parsley, mushrooms, carrots, beet tops, dandelion greens, cucumbers, and nuts.

9. *Phosphorus* aids in the assimilation of calcium, provides

our bones with strength and rigidity, promotes digestion, and nourishes the brain and nerves. The more we think, the more we need phosphorus. We could not live without it. A lack of phosphorus is shown by fatigue, tiredness, and anemia. In its inorganic state it is also a hard poison, but when organized by the vegetable kingdom it becomes suitable and very useful for the building and maintenance of the body. It also is needed in the formation of good blood. Supply the need by foods rich in phosphorus such as (fruits) cherries, huckleberries, blackberries, black Mission figs, oranges, limes, and white figs, and (vegetables) lettuce, celery, onions, spinach, kale, radishes, carrots, and Brussels sprouts.

10. *Sulphur* is a constituent of the hair and nails. An anti poison, a blood purifier, a nerve tonic, a system stimulator by acting on every cell in the body, it activates the muscles, energizes the liver, and increases the bile flow. It is not only a purifier, but a beautifier of the whole body. Sulphur should be taken uncooked; cooked sulphur may have destructive effects, causing biliousness or gas trouble. Supply the need from sulphur-rich foods such as (vegetables) raw onions, garlic, cabbage, radishes, horseradish, turnips, chives, cauliflower, kale, sorrel, and Brussels sprouts, and (fruits) cranberries, currants, raspberries, pineapples, Brazil nuts, and filberts.

11. *Potassium* is a blood and bone builder, a nourisher of the cell life of the whole body. Potassium is the chief alkaline-producing agent in the body, reacting against body acids by sup plying alkaline properties to the blood and tissues. It purifies the blood, heals wounds, and nourishes the glands. Lack of it means constipation, weakness, and a general run-down condition. Supply the need from potassium-rich foods such as (vegetables) carrots, lettuce, raw cabbage, parsley, onions, beets, spin ach, cauliflower, leeks, garlic, and raw potatoes, and (fruits) strawberries, blackberries, huckleberries, cherries, apples, pears, peaches, prunes, plums, grapes, figs, dates, and bananas.

12. *Magnesium* keeps body and brain cool; it prevents the brain from becoming inflamed from excitement or emotion. It

is called the "fan belt" for the brain. It neutralizes abnormal acid conditions of the body. It aids in forming blood and bones. It is considered, with calcium, the base of the bones, and it is an ingredient for the natural functioning of the bowels. Supply the need from magnesium-rich foods such as (vegetables) lettuce, celery, cucumbers, carrots, dandelions, asparagus, tomatoes, spinach, kale, onions, garlic, and leeks; (fruits) apples, oranges, grapefruit, lemons, limes, peaches, grapes, prunes, plums, blackberries, and cherries; and (nuts) Brazil nuts, pecans, piñons, walnuts, hazelnuts, cashew, and almonds.

13. *Iron* is very important. It is a complicated compound containing 2,000 atoms to a molecule. Only the vegetable king dom can produce this highly complex element. Iron carries oxygen to all parts of the body. It is a magnet for the attraction of oxygen. The more iron one has in one's system, the more oxygen one can consume, and the more life and vitality one will have. Iron, therefore, means life, health, efficiency, and vitality. But only organic iron is man's best friend. Inorganic iron is an irritant to the kidneys and cannot be assimilated by the body. Iron deficiency means disease, particularly anemia, and depression and unhappiness. Supply the need with good foods rich in iron, such as (vegetables) lettuce, spinach, celery, green beans, green peas, all dark-green, leafy vegetables, carrots, turnips, asparagus, leeks, onions, and radishes; (fruits) apricots, apples, pears, grapes, raisins, figs, prunes, plums, cherries, blue berries, raspberries, and huckleberries; and nuts of all kinds. Milk supplies no iron.

14. *Silicon* is the needed material to build the skin, the hair, and the nails, and also the covering of various organs like the brain. It is a stabilizer of the muscles and an antiseptic. It keeps the blood warm and makes the hair shiny. It is needed for the vascular system, and gives strength and vigor to the whole body. Silicon is found in the outer layer of fruits and vegetables, there fore do not throw them away; use them. Lack of silicon means exhaustion and low endurance. Supply the need from silicon-rich foods such as (vegetables) cucumbers, lettuce, parsnips,

asparagus tips, beet tops, green peppers, radishes, spinach, watercress, and okra, and (fruits) watermelon, apples, peaches, grapes, cherries, figs, dates, and raisins.

15. *Manganese* is the stabilizer of the nerves. Lack of it means confusion of mind and worry. It gives nourishment to the generative organs and the various glands. It also serves the outer covering of the bones. It gives strength and elasticity to the body. Supply the need from manganese-rich foods such as (vegetables) watercress, endive, lettuce, celery, parsley, beets, cucumbers, dandelions, mint, soy beans, brown rice; (fruits) apricots, and prunes; and nuts of all kinds.

16. *Iodine* is the defender and protector of the brain and the nervous system, the regulator of metabolism, and the helpmate and strengthener of the glands and reproductive functions of the body. It is also the equalizer of arterial pressure. Lack of it means goitre, nervousness, uneven pulse palpitation, and excitability. Supply the need from good iodine-rich foods such as (vegetables) sea kelp, sea dulse, sea lettuce, onions, garlic, tomatoes, carrots, mushrooms, and artichokes, and (fruits) apples, pears, pineapples, grapes, and orange juice. Use only organic iodine, which is obtainable through the vegetable kingdom.

These are the food elements, and their sources of supply, that correspond to the sixteen elements the body is made of. As it is impossible to build buildings, boats, bridges, and so on, without the right material and a sufficient quantity of it, it is likewise impossible to build a physical personality without the proper material and the correct amount. As remarked before, seventy million Americans are deficient in one kind or another of these elements. Would this not also indicate a deficiency in knowledge of what to eat and of how to eat?

8. THE TRANSFORMATION OF FOOD INTO A BODY

THE TRANSFORMATION of food into a body, or how a body is built from food, is indeed an amazing, highly interesting, and wonderful story. A whole book could be written on this really fascinating topic. But in our personality engineering we must be satisfied with just a short chapter and some highlights. Health-food centers throughout the country carry a good selection of books on this subject. Some are very interesting and read like a novel. There is a saying that is indeed true: "We are what we eat, and what we eat today will walk and talk tomorrow."

Take a good look at the food upon your table, and imagine the tremendous changes that food will undergo within you after it enters your mouth. In a very short period of time that food will see and hear, walk and talk, love or hate, make you strong or weak, ugly or beautiful. Yes, that very food you eat becomes protoplasm; it builds the cells whereby your eyes see and your ears hear; it nourishes your brain cells so that you can think and plan.

Will it be worth your while to study, consider, and select for your eating pleasure these foods that have real nutritional value? Have you ever given real thought and consideration to what the food you eat can do and will do for you and your personality? And what a tremendous, indeed awful, transformation the food you eat must undergo in your body to accomplish all this?

HOW   IS   IT   DONE?

Science tells us that our bodies are composed of about 30 trillion cells. That most of these perish within the course of a year and must be replaced continually (metabolism). Dr. Brown tells us that approximately one trillion hemoglobin cells perish every hour, all of which must be replaced. Thus the need and demand of the body for new cells is tremendous. It is estimated that in a normal body 18,000 new body and hemoglobin cells are created or manufactured every second around the clock, or 1,080,000 every minute, 64,800,000 every hour, 1,555,200,000 every day. What a terrific job! To do this tremendous work right, the body depends on you and your discriminating, careful selection of food. There are approximately 30 trillion cells that must be fed regularly with the right kind of food, says Dr. Brown. If we fail the body in this tremendous responsibility, that is, eat and drink indiscriminately, the result will be detrimental. And as a nation it seems we do this very thing. We shamefully fail our bodies in this great task.

In *Overfed and Undernourished*, Dr. H. Curtis Wood, Jr., tells us that in 1957, in the seven thousand hospitals of the United States, eight million operations were performed. The number of patients is given as 91,800,000 for the same period. They spent $13,500,000,000 for medical services. And the major cause for so much ill health is to be found in wrong eating habits, states another authority. Does this not reveal an appalling, a frightful lack of understanding of the all important science of nutrition—of how a body is built from food?

Let us follow the food from the table until it is ready to be used by the body to build eyes that can see, and ears that can hear.

First, when selecting food, remember that the food you eat must contain all the material the cells are made of. The components must include the three basic elements, protein, carbohydrates, and fats plus the minerals and vitamins.

Second, the body is unable to use the food in the form it enters the mouth. It must continually undergo many changes until it can be used by the body, either as building blocks or as combustion (energy) material.

Protein is all the nitrogenous foods known as C.O.H.N.P.S.

Blood plasma corresponds to the building blocks of the body, C.O.H.N.P.S.

Carbohydrates are the starchy and sugary foods, C.O.H.

Hydrocarbon represents the fats and oils, C.H.

It is interesting to note that the protein upon the table and the blood plasma in our bodies correspond exactly in formula. But if we should inspect the blood plasma under the microscope and view the protein upon the table we would be unable to find any resemblance or points of likeness at all. Blood plasma is the final protein material in the body for building, rejuvenating, and maintaining the body cells. The great difference in appearance can be compared with that of a piece of black coal and a beautiful, sparkling diamond. Both are almost pure carbon, but what a difference between the piece of coal and the brilliant, shining diamond! The great difference between the protein in the food upon the table and the protein in the blood plasma is a similar one.

Before we consider how these changes in food take place, let us take one more look at the carbohydrates and the hydrocarbons. Note that they are minus the "N" that stands for the element nitrogen. We know that the Creator in His wisdom included in our economy the protective element nitrogen, for without it we would burn up and could not exist. Since these two parts of our food, carbohydrates and hydrocarbons (starchy and sugary foods and oils), have no protective nitrogen in their components, they cannot exist; they are being burned up, and become ashes.

Again I would like to drive home the point that we as a nation live too much on starches, sugar, and fats, which are detrimental to our health and quite useless in the building of vibrant, vigorous, physical personalities. We need only small amounts of sugar and fat, but we need *protein* for building the *body*, and protein with the *life* principle, not dead, decaying protein, if we figure protein a first-class product, not a second-class one from the remains of dead animals.

Now let us follow the food to see how the changes in the

body are wrought. The process is divided into four stages, in-gestion, digestion, absorption, and metabolism.

Ingestion is the introduction of food into the body.

Digestion is the conversion of food into a state of readiness for use by the body. It is divided into three stages: salivary, stomach, and intestinal digestion.

Absorption is the sucking up of the prepared food into the blood stream, called, professionally, osmosis.

Metabolism is what happens to the food after absorption. It denotes the chemical changes that take place constantly, and are necessary when food is assimilated into the tissues, creating new cells and maintaining, or feeding, old ones.

Thirty trillion body cells! Naturally they must be very small. They are just one eight-thousandth of an inch in diameter, but they are completely organized units. They could rightly be called living creatures. They live and work; they can get sick and die. You will agree that one eight-thousandth of an inch in diameter is not very big, therefore it follows that these tiny cells cannot swallow anything but infinitesimal atoms. And these are what the body has to prepare out of that coarse protein we eat.

The large bites of food and the large molecules, which make up the different kinds of nutritious substances, must be broken down into ever smaller, yes, infinitesimally small, proportions.

The work starts in the mouth, where we have three sets of salivary glands. You may be surprised at the work they do. They produce as much saliva as a fresh milking goat gives milk, three or four quarts every day, or about one thousand quarts of saliva each year. This digestive salivary fluid is alkaline, and consists of water, minerals, salts, and two enzymes called amylase and maltase. They are concerned with carbohydrate digestion, in breaking down starchy foods into maltose sugars.

You probably have had some mouth-watering experiences. Your eyes beheld and your sense of smell perceived the odor of some succulent food, ready and good to eat—and what happened? Your salivary glands in your mouth went into action immediately, producing an extra-large amount of saliva in anticipation and expectation of the good pleasures to come. There is a reason for this phenomenon.

When your eyes have selected the food you want to eat immediately, the subconscious mind (henceforth called the H.Q.) gives an order to the salivary glands (they are the receptionists for the food trains): "Get ready! Food is on its way!"

SALIVARY DIGESTION AND MASTICATION

When the food enters the mouth, it receives a cheerful reception. It was expected, and everything is in readiness. Immediately, it is bathed, massaged, softened, and lubricated by the saliva. This is called salivary digestion. The saliva starts to change the starch into dextrose sugar. This is the sugar that is found in dates, grapes, figs, prunes and other sweet fruits, but it is not the same as commercial white sugar. Simultaneously, the teeth must cut and grind the food into the smallest particles, and, using about sixty muscles, mix the food and saliva together. The whole process is called mastication. When this is well done, we are then ready for the next step.

SWALLOWING

The ball, or bolus, of food is gently but surely forced by little policemen (small muscles) down the esophagus, a tube about ten inches long that connects the mouth with the stomach. These little policemen are rather strong. They have orders from the H.Q. for one-way traffic only, and they will do their work faithfully, even under adverse circumstances. You may even stand on your head and eat something. They will then have to work the food uphill, but they will surely do it. They have been ordered by the H.Q. to convey the food to the stomach, and there it will go, whether they have to force it up or down. You do not have to think about the direction in which the food shall go, down or up. It's the H.Q.'s business to get the food to the second station for further processing, and if you don't interfere your H.Q. will do the work well and satisfactorily. Now the food is ready for the next step.

CHURNING

The stomach is a muscular bag that normally holds between two and two and a half quarts of food. It is lined with a membrane varying from one eighth to one fourth of an inch in thickness, and is filled with several thousand tiny gastric glands that produce from four to five quarts of gastric juice daily, or about 1,800 quarts, or 3,600 pounds, annually. When the food enters the mouth, the H.Q. immediately wires the stomach and the gastric glands: "Food is on its way! Get ready!" Immediately they obey. They get the gastric juice ready, which is acid, the opposite of the salivary juice, which is alkaline. The component parts of the gastric juice are hydrochloric acid and two enzymes, pepsin for the digestion of protein, and lipase for acting on emulsified fats. Babies have a third enzyme, rennin, for the digestion of milk.

The gastric juice of adults lacks this third enzyme, rennin, or it is inactive at the pH of the gastric content of the normal adult. For that reason adults cannot digest milk completely. It remains as mucus, a gummy-like substance, clogging the system. More than 30 million Americans suffer annually from so-called common colds, often several times during the year. What causes them? Many doctors believe that partly digested milk is the culprit. When food enters the stomach, the thousands of gastric glands pour the gastric juice into the food, and the stomach at once begins to contract and expand, squeezing, mixing, and churning the food.

Slight muscular waves start from the upper end of the stomach and move toward the lower end. Each wave takes forty seconds to traverse the distance, but every tenth second starts a new wave, causing three waves simultaneously to move across the stomach. Over 2,100 such waves pass over the stomach per hour. Besides this, there are movements from side to side. This churning action reduces the content of the stomach to a milk-like emulsion called chyme.

As soon as the contents of the stomach are thoroughly mixed, which takes from one to five hours, depending on the kind and amount of food eaten, the chyme is allowed to pass through the lower stomach gate, called the pyloric valve, into the duodenum, often referred to as the second stomach. In fact, it is the upper part of the so-called small intestine.

Let me remind you that each station has its specific work to do in this great task of changing food into a wonderful physical personality. One station cannot do the work for any of the others.

Consciously, we have something to do with the food in the first station, the mouth. After the food has passed the esophagus, however, it is no longer under the control of the objective conscious mind; it is beyond conscious consideration. The subconscious mind completely takes charge from there on, and handles the work through the involuntary nervous system. It is that part of our being that is involuntarily under the direct control of our Creator.

So we see that the building and maintaining of the physical personality still is on a co-operative basis with the Creator. Whether you believe or not, whether you are willing or not willing to co-operate with the great "I AM," you will have to realize that He has not granted you authority over many things of the great unknown within you.

You have no authority over the food after it passes the esophagus. You have no authority over the air after it passes into the lungs. You have only partial control over your breathing, and thank the Lord for it, for by your forgetfulness you might not be here today. You have no control over the beating of your heart, over the work of your glands, over the delicate machinery of your physical body, or life itself. But the Creator has granted his human beings the role of assistants by giving them free will in two things: in selecting healthful food to eat; and in chewing and masticating the food thoroughly.

And remember this: salivary digestion, changing the starch into dextrose, can only be done in the mouth by the alkaline saliva, and the amylopin in the small intestine. It cannot be done in the stomach, by the gastric juices.

Therefore, in physical personality engineering it is imperative to pay attention to the proper mastication of the food eaten, in cutting, grinding, and mixing the food with saliva. I can assure you that there are no teeth in the stomach, nor any alkaline salivary glands to take care of the starchy foods you have eaten. The H. Q. asks your co-operation in this matter of cutting, grinding, and thoroughly mixing the food with saliva, and if you do not fail in this digesting job, the H.Q. promises you that it will not fail you the rest of the way. Now let us see what happens to the food that we left in the upper small intestine, the duodenum.

INTESTINAL   DIGESTION

Many people have a notion that the stomach is the main organ of digestion, and believe that as soon as food enters the stomach it is turned immediately into blood and energy. That is not so. The stomach only prepares the food for actual digestion, which takes place in the small intestine.

The pulpy mass, the chyme, undergoes further elaboration by the peristaltic action of the small intestine, which mixes it with the juice of two large glands, the liver and the pancreas. Here in the small intestine the digestion of all classes of food will be completed.

The liver, the largest gland in our body, does the most gigantic manufacturing job, considering its size, in all the world. This organ is a marvelous laboratory manned by fifteen to thirty million little chemists (hepatic cells) that could teach our most learned chemists many secrets about their profession. To study the story and the work of the liver is a fascinating one, but in our study of the digestion and preparation of food for absorption, we only can point out the fact that the liver manufactures about three or four pounds of bile daily, or somewhat more than one thousand pounds a year. When the chyme arrives in the duodenum, bile is poured into the food immediately, enabling the digestion of fats, which are broken down into fatty acids and glycerol. The small globules are known as emulsion, which can be absorbed.

The bile also neutralizes the chyme, which we learned was acid by the presence of gastric juice from the stomach, and this acid would hinder further digestion. Through the action of bile and pancreatic juice the food now again is made alkaline. The pancreas also manufactures about three or four pounds of pancreatic juice daily, or about a half ton a year, and pours it into the chyme. To these digestive juices are added nine more enzymes, which have the ability to act as little hatchets. They split the food into smaller and still smaller particles as it travels along the twenty- to twenty-five-foot length of the intestines. Thus the final stage for the digestion is set.

Let us take one more look at the all important protein for our building program. The digestive juices have broken down the protein into proteose and then converted it into peptones. This is the name for the soluble protein. Now an enzyme from the pancreas called erepsin performs the most important job of changing the peptones into the all important amino acids, the real building blocks.

In the tissues, the wear and tear of the muscles must be replaced by these amino acids. They are indispensable in the growing, building, and maintaining of the human body. The original food from the table is now completely reduced to a liquid called chyle and is ready for absorption.

ABSORPTION

Absorption involves the selective permeability of the cells as well as the physical process of diffusion and osmosis. This takes place in the small intestine. For this reason some writers call the small intestine the body's dining hall. Dr. Brown elaborates very fittingly on the absorption, or osmosis, as the loading of a moving cafeteria train. How is it done?

The wall of the twenty-five-foot-long small intestine is fitted with a sponge-like membrane that contains about ten million hairlike filaments, or fingerlike projections, called villi. These villis act as little suction pumps. Along with the small intestine runs a system of lymphatic vessels. They collect the prepared fatty acid and the glycerol, transporting them by way of the veins into the blood stream.

The carbohydrates and amino acids are collected by the portal circulation and carried into the liver. The blood, with all the nutrients, gets its final inspection, and is filtered. A part of the glucose (sugar) is stored as glycogen for later use for heat and energy. The amino acid, minerals, and vitamins are also carried by the blood plasma to the tissues. They are ready for the assembly job, and are rushed to wherever the need is greatest. What is left in this amazing food story and feeding system is metabolism.

METABOLISM

The cells of the tissues of the human body are constantly undergoing chemical changes. These changes constitute what is generally spoken of as a building up of cells known as anabolism and a breaking down of cells known as catabolism, the whole process being included in the term metabolism. The broken-down cells are carried by the blood plasma back to the liver, which reuses the material to make more bile.

Dr. Brown gives a short review of the process as follows:

After the absorption the moving cafeteria system works beautifully. While not literally true, it may be imagined that the tiny bundles of various food elements are laid out in an orderly fashion along the edges of the flat cars which make up the train.

Sugars and starches have become simple sugars.

Fats have become glycerine and fatty acids.

Proteins have been broken up into forms of amino acids, and certain mineral salts.

The fatty acids and glycerol are carried away as chyle (name of the final emulsion in the intestine) to little tubes known as lacteals of the lymphatic system and into the general circulation.

The sugars and amino acids are hustled into a large vein, the portal vein, and carried to the liver for inspection, purification or storage.

When the full train leaves the union station, which we will call the heart, it is traveling very rapidly—thirty feet per second. This is much too fast for the tiny cells to grab their food, so that it is necessary to slow down the rate of traveling.

In the smallest tubes, the capillaries and lymph channels, where the food is extracted, the train moves one inch a minute. The hungry cells have plenty time to select their meals, and if they wish to smack their imaginary lips.

This, in short, is the amazing story of how food is transformed into a body, and a body built from food. Now let us learn the moral of the story.

A NIGHTMARE IN A STOMACH

*(An allegorical conversation between a stomach, a
peptic gland, and a gastric gland)*

"It's terrible! It's terrible! Oh, it's terrible!" groaned the old stomach. "But what can I do? What can I do? I worked for six hours as hard as I could, and the gastric juice dissolved everything possible, but I cannot get that old stuff out, and it is getting harder and harder all the time. The old gateman pylorus will not open the door and let the stuff out.

"Of course, I understand it is the imperative business of the old fellow to keep the orifice shut tight against everything but pure chyme. Certainly this stuff is not ready yet for the duodenum, and perhaps never will be. Oh, it's terrible! What shall I do?"

"Good morning," said the peptic gland to the gastric lipase gland.

"Good morning," replied the other as both got ready for the new day's work. "I just hope that our dear old faithful stomach will not have such hard work, and so much trouble, as he had yesterday/"

"Yes, indeed," rejoined the peptic gland. "He was so exhausted last night, when the last bit of chyme squeezed through the pylorus, that I am sure he couldn't have contracted one single time more, no matter what the old master would have sent down."

"And the worst of it is," submitted the gastric gland, "there is a wretched residue of indigestible stuff that just cannot get through the pylorus at all. And that stuff has been there all night and is hard already. It is fermenting and disintegrating. It stinks already like that old stuff in the colon."

"Yes," said the peptic gland, "it's all on account of that old beefsteak, with all that hot sauce, pepper, and salty pickles. That stuff killed some of my sisters and brothers outright."

"And believe it or not, on top of all this the master sent down very hot tea, and ice cream, and beer, and whatnot. I just wondered if our master was out to commit suicide," said the gastric gland.

"It's too bad, too bad," said the peptic gland. "If the master will not treat our good old stomach any better, he will surely get sick and die. And then they will carry him out of his nice home-feet first."

This parable is only too true in many cases. A prominent Vienna doctor estimates that more than 80 per cent of adults at present are suffering with prolapsed, or out of shape, stomachs, the majority because of careless eating.

THE MORAL OF THE STORY

If we conform to nature's laws, all will be well with the transformation of the right food we eat into a beautiful body, full of vigor and life, the right foundation for a perfect per-sonality—body, soul, and spirit.

But the food and the eating habits of today are such that

they well may destroy the very foundation for such a perfect personality.

Tea or coffee is served with meals, a common, bad habit from coast to coast. These beverages are not food but narcotics, destroying the very process of digestion. And remember, it is not the *food you eat* that builds your physical personality, but the *food that is digested.* Any liquid with meals weakens the digestion, dilutes the digestive fluid. But tea and coffee destroy it, rendering other foods indigestible.

If you doubt the above statement, try it out for yourself. Here is an experiment. Make a good strong brew of tea, just as you like it, but don't drink it, pour it over your favorite piece of beefsteak and let it soak for half an hour in the tea. Then see what happens! Don't be surprised to find that the beefsteak has become as black as coal and as hard as sole leather. Why? Because tea contains tannin.

You cook the beefsteak on an iron grill; the beefsteak itself has some iron. Mix iron and tannin together and you have a combination that makes ink. Stir your cup of tea with an iron spoon. You don't have to wait very long before you have not tea but ink to drink.

Hard as sole leather? Yes. Leather is made by soaking the animal hide in a solution of tannin. So when one eats a piece of beefsteak or other meat and drinks a cup of strong tea with it, the tannic acid combines with the connective tissues of the meat and it becomes leather in the stomach. Truly, if you understand the working of your digestion, you will easily understand what a terrible influence such a combination will have upon the digestive process. You will have this combination in your stomach, not for an hour, but for five hours or more. Nor is this all!

The theine of the tea plant is an alkaloid with as powerful a toxic effect on animals and man as strychnine and morphine. Each pound of tea contains 224 grains of theine, which science considers to be the same as caffeine. Seven grains will kill a cat or a rabbit, or any animal of that size. One grain will kill a frog.

When a person eats a beefsteak and drinks a cup of coffee

or tea with it, not digestion, but the leather-making process, starts in the stomach. Theine paralyzes the salivary glands, thus hindering the flow of the saliva and the digestion of other foods, such as bread, noodles, vegetables, and cake.

Tea and coffee drinking have become a national curse. That paralyzing effect starts in the mouth and goes through to the colon, with indigestion, autointoxication, and constipation, along with all the connecting pains and nightmares, following it.

Another bad habit is that of making food "hot" or "fiery" with irritating spices like pepper, mustard, sharp vinegar, or pickles, which irritate the mucus membrane of the whole digestive system, mouth, stomach, small intestine, and large intestine. Naturally, if hot spices are used, it is no wonder that there is a greater demand for water or liquid. One evil never comes alone.

When I was a teen-ager, I followed the common practice. I ate meat, bacon, and so on, and used to handle the pepper and salt shakers like anyone twice or three times my age. When I was nineteen years old I received wonderful lessons on healthful living. Immediately I stopped that senseless seasoning, and there I learned a lesson for life. Only nineteen years old, and all the fine taste buds on the surface of my tongue burned and gone. What about my stomach and intestines? They had their share too, but I did not realize it. The hot condiments had taken care of that. For more than a quarter of a year I had no taste whatever. I could not differentiate between noodles or shoestrings. Today, I very seldom use a salt shaker and no hot spices are used in our kitchen. I enjoy with full pleasure the fine and delicious natural foods on our table, simple but tasty without the hot spices. Learn your lesson here; I had to pay the price.

In a medical book I found this sentence, which gives some food for thought: "Very few people die—most of them don't wait for the time, but kill themselves."

9. ENZYMES

What are enzymes?

Enzymes are catalytic agents of a protein nature. They are manufactured by specialized living cells.

What is their work?

They are ordered to produce chemical changes in certain other substances.

They are very powerful in their action, for a very small amount can accomplish great and very difficult changes.

They change other substances without undergoing any changes themselves.

They are specialists; they can act only on the substance for which they are appointed. An enzyme working on carbohydrates cannot work on protein. An enzyme working in an alkaline medium cannot work in acid fluid, and vice versa.

The enzymes of digestion.

There are fifteen known enzymes engaged in the digestive process: in salivary digestion, two work in an alkaline medium; in gastric digestion, three work in an acid medium; and in intestinal digestion ten work in an alkaline medium. In the large intestine the medium is an acid one.

FLESH EATING VERSUS VEGETARIANISM AND PERSONALITY

Man is a carnivorous production,
And must have meals, at least one meal a day;
He cannot live, like woodcocks, upon suction,
But, like the shark and tiger, must have prey.

> Although his anatomical construction
> Bears vegetables, in a grumbling way
> You laboring people think beyond all question
> Beef, veal, and mutton better for digestion.
>
> LORD BYRON, *Don Juan*

Since the days of Pythagoras and Hippocrates, more than 2,000 years ago, down to the present, it has been a much debated question whether a vegetable or a meat diet was best and right for man. In the above stanzas from Don Juan, Byron calls man a flesh eater, a "carnivorous production" whereas his construction calls for a vegetarian diet.

In passionate disputes, pro and con, strong arguments have been brought into the fight on both sides. Dr. M. O. Garten says in *The Cycle of Health:*

> The ingestion of flesh foods of any type is not as ideal as assumed by the average person. There have been many arguments for and against meat eating on various different grounds, such as the aesthetic, economic, therapeutic, etc.
>
> The vegetarian claims that the fleshless diet is far superior, a conception which should deserve particular emphasis in regard to rearing children and in case of illness. Vegetarianism provides, without a doubt, the most ideal and perfect diet not only in overcoming but also in the prevention of disease. Children, therefore, should never accustom themselves to the taste of meats, in order to develop strong minds and bodies, as well as immunity to disease. When children grow up in this manner they will always prefer vegetable foods because they will thoroughly enjoy them and consider flesh foods distasteful, if not repulsive.

Dr. Clem Davis, in Divine Diet, challenges with these words:

> If you fear that a meatless diet would make the mind less keen, the following list of outstanding personalities from the world's honor roll gives a strong argument in its favor: Plato, Ovid and Buddha, Leonardo da Vinci, John Wesley, Swedenborg, Shelley, Thoreau, Benjamin Franklin, Tolstoy, Gandhi, George Bernard Shaw—all those, and many, many others were strict vegetarians.

We all stand aghast at the ills of mankind. Whether they are the result of the meat diet is yet to be proved, but the evidences are overwhelming that our manner of living is killing us too young and too fast. I firmly believe that every energy, flavor and cleanser can be found in the vegetable kingdom. Every individual must make his own choice for better or worse. If you feel a revulsion against meat diets, it is high time you switched to the vegetable kingdom.

Diet should produce physical strength and an alert mind, a trim and well formed body, an optimistic outlook, active ambition, a general sense of well-being and peace of mind. If your present diet is not producing these results, it is high time you change it to find the correct and desired attributes.

E. G. White, the great health reformer, in *Fundamentals· of Christian Education*, classifies flesh foods with harmful and intoxicating commodities:

> Let every one resist the temptation to use wine, tobacco, flesh meats, tea and coffee. Experience has demonstrated that far better work can be accomplished without these harmful things.

Proponents of a meat diet or a mixed diet contend that flesh foods contain the best protein and an appreciable amount of amino acids, minerals, and fats. In an earlier chapter we stated that the Creator has taken good care of our need for protein and amino acids, minerals and vitamins, in the vegetable kingdom, and that flesh protein is lifeless, secondhand protein, which God only permitted as an emergency measure after the Great Deluge. In the world of today, there are other emergencies in which a meat diet may be found necessary.

I have often traveled on the roof of the world, in Tibet. The Tibetans live at a high altitude, from 12,000 to 17,000 feet above sea level. When traveling at such high altitudes we kept to a vegetarian diet, but we had to carry our food supply with us from the lowlands, since the foods were not available at such an altitude. I well remember one incident.

I was traveling with Dr. John Nevins Andrews, superintendent of the Tibetan Mission Hospital at Tatsienlu, which is one of the gateways from China to Tibet. We were ten days' traveling distance from the hospital, camping at a large settlement beside a lamasery. A man approached us and begged the doctor for help. One of the outstanding character traits of the Tibetans is their great physical courage, which showed in this man. He suffered from dropsy. The accumulation of water in the abdominal cavity was tremendous. I had never seen anything like it. That he lived at all was a marvel to us.

He said about this: "Please, doctor, help me! I have not seen my feet for a long time. I cannot bow, and I feel very uncomfortable. Will you please cut me open and look into my stomach, and see what is the trouble?" The doctor did help him, and relieved him of several gallons of water.

He was a high Tibetan official, and very grateful for the help he received. In appreciation, he, the lamasery, and the settlement gave us a royal dinner. At that dinner sixteen different kinds of meat dishes were served, including snake meat from an Indian boa. That was the only time in my life that snake meat has been offered to me. It smelled very sweet and looked as white as bleached sugar, whiter even than pork. How did it taste? I do not know, for all I ate at that dinner was half a bowl of white rice. That is all I got, because rice was the most precious commodity they could offer. It had to be carried up from the lowlands of either China or India, hundreds of miles over steep and high mountains, on the backs of human carriers.

Though I did not partake of any of the meat dishes, for the people, living at that high altitude, meat was the only food available 365 days a year. Besides some alpine grass for the wild life and the domestic yak (the Tibetan cow), there is absolutely no vegetation to be found, no grains, no vegetables, no fruits. Once, on the south side of a mountain slope, at 14,000 feet, I found some fir and pine groves inhabited by black bears, but such an exception proves the rule.

What is true for people living at such an extreme altitude is equally true for those living in an extreme latitude, like the Lapps and the Eskimos, who live nearest to the North Pole.

What is inevitable and cannot be prevented in these remote regions, where people unfortunately have to live and therefore have no other choice, should not necessarily hold true for those living in more favorable places on earth. These are emergency cases, comparable to the time after the Great Deluge, when all vegetation was destroyed. God then permitted, as an emergency measure, the consumption of meat in a restricted manner. He divided the animals into two classes: the clean and the unclean. The clean were allowed and the unclean forbidden. But today, even the animals that were then called clean are not in a healthy state; they carry disease and seldom are fit even as secondary food. E. G. White says:

> Could you know just the nature of the meat you eat, could you see the animals when living from which the flesh is taken when dead, you would turn with loathing from your flesh meats. The very animals whose flesh you eat are frequently so diseased that, if left alone, they would die of themselves; but while the breath of life is still in them, they are killed and brought to market. You take direct into your system poisons of the worst kind, and yet you realize it not.

In 1943, during those dreadful days of the Second World War, I was carried on a stretcher into a hospital, in Hankow, Central China. I was unable to walk; my knees were swollen and stiff, the arthritic pain unbearable. The doctors were not sure of the cause of it, and for relief gave me what then and there was available—some salicylic acid shots (a salt solution used in the treatment of rheumatism). To their amazement, within two days I walked home like a spring chicken. But after four weeks I had to go through the same experience again, and it then became a regular occurrence every three or four weeks.

"We cannot go on this way or we soon will have you on the operating table," said the doctor, and he insisted on my going to Shanghai for a thorough blood test and checkup.

In Shanghai, the doctor said: "No, if you had not listened to your doctor, he would not have had you on the operating table, but in a coffin." Ptomaine poisoning was the verdict. The word ptomaine comes from the Greek *ptoma*, meaning corpse, and is derived from putrefying and decomposing dead protein, generally from decaying animal protein such as meat or fish. In my case it did not come from eating meat or fish, because I had not eaten any, but from a tooth, decaying under a gold crown and sending the ptomaine poison directly into my blood stream, which caused the swelling, stiffness, and pain. The culprit was pulled out, and never since have I experienced any trouble.

I relate this experience for a purpose. There are hundreds of thousands of sufferers from rheumatic and arthritic pains, with stiff, swollen, and deformed limbs. My experience may give them something to think about. Could decaying animal protein in the intestines be one or even the cause of their affliction? Many doctors believe just that. Here is what Dr. N. W. Walker has to say about it:

> Physiologically, the eating of meat increases the acidity of the body. In the processes of digestion and in breaking down the meat into its original amino acids, a vast amount of uric acid is generated in the body. If the body could eliminate this immediately, it might do only little harm. But actually what happens is that the muscles absorb enormous amounts of the uric acid, and in the course of time they are thoroughly saturated with it. Eventually this acid forms into crystals with sharp needlelike points, which cause the pain and discomfort known as rheumatism, arthritis, neuritis, sciatica, nephritis (Bright's disease), and some diseases of the liver.

The preference and popularity of a meat diet is defended mainly because of the tasty flavor of properly cooked flesh foods. But after all, flesh foods of any kind are not as ideal as many assume. Many people are ruled by appetite; this is a liability. Principle should rule and not appetite. E. G. White says:

> Eating merrily to please the appetite is a transgression of nature's laws.
> If the appetite is allowed to rule, the mind will be brought under its control. One of the strongest temptations that man has to meet is upon the point of appetite, and those who are slaves to appetite will fail in perfecting a Christian character.

It has been reported that "out of 158 Bulgarian centenarians, 118 lived strictly on vegetable food, 5 on a meat diet, and 35 on a mixed diet." This should settle any argument over which diet is to be preferred in personality engineering, and in seeking youthfulness and longevity. A meat diet shortens life and makes for misery.

Biblical history records that the patriarchs who never touched meat for food lived 900 years or more. Noah, the last of them, lived to be 950 years old, but Noah's sons, the first generation of meat eaters after the Flood, only lived about 600 years. Meat eating had shortened their lives by one third of the possible span. It shortened life in those days, and the Bulgarian Research Committee shows that it has done so through the ages and still does today.

A poem entitled "The Choice of Food" by Maggie C. Richardson, quoted in the Diet System, is appropriated here:

> Then, what shall we eat to keep disease away?
> Is the question we encounter day by day.
>
> This question worth is of careful thought,
> For health cannot be hired, sold or bought.
>
> Let's choose the food that makes the better health,
> Which is of greater worth than all our wealth.
>
> Let's choose the food our MAKER gave to man
> While still he lived according to His plan,
>
> That food God gave to him in days of yore,
> So that he lived nine hundred years or more.
>
> Meat is an unscientific food for man.
> Meat is an uneconomical food for man.

The land and the food consumed by the 25,000,000 head of livestock in this country would support 500,000,000 human beings.

10. OBESITY AND PERSONALITY

THE GREATEST obstacle to be surmounted in building a perfect physical personality, keeping youthful, and obtaining longevity is ignorance concerning what to eat and how to eat for health. The great majority of people transgress natural laws every time they sit down to eat. The body is loaded, even overloaded, with "foodless foods" that not only have little or no value, but the effects of which are harmful and detrimental to the inner system and the whole body. Thus great numbers of people impair, mar, and disfigure their physical personality and become chronic invalids just because of thoughtlessness in eating. The fact that more than 41,000,000 Americans suffer from obesity, and spend more than $250,000,000 each year for reducing pills and in slimming salons is alarming and eye-opening. What is the reason? Why sacrifice the graceful lines of waist, chest, bust, and limbs, and lose the charm and poise of personality? There may be a few minor reasons, but the main reason is *gratification of the appetite.*

There are a few minor causes for overweight, but the major one is the ingestion of more food than the body needs or can use in its work. Overeating is the compulsive force that drives away youth and youthfulness, and invites a host of diseases, premature old age, senility, and untimely death. This is confirmed by one of the leading life insurance companies. Its records show that people between the ages of 30 and 45 whose weight is fifty pounds or more above normal for their age group have an above-normal death rate: from heart disease, it is 200 per cent; from apoplexy, 200 per cent; from cirrhosis of the liver, 300 per cent; from diabetes, 400 per cent; and from other diseases between 200 and 250 per cent. The close relation between overweight and shortening of life is thus obvious.

The *Medical and Health Encyclopedia*, edited by Dr. Morris Fishbein, makes this contribution to the subject:

Excess weight can be associated with shortness of breath, increased tendency of fatigue, trouble with the joints, increased failure of the heart, damage to other vital organs. People with obesity get diabetes more often than those of ordinary weight. Most fat people, though they do not admit it, simply love to eat, and if they do not eat much at meals, they begin taking extra food in small amounts all through the day and before going to bed at night. These habits must be broken.

Overeating is dangerous. Aside from the unsightliness of the ugly surplus fat, a portion of the excess food will crystallize, pass into the blood, and be deposited along the mucus surface of the arteries. The result may be arterio-sclerosis, or hardening of the arteries. If deposited elsewhere it may result in stiffness in the joints, arthritis, rheumatism, gout, lumbago, or whatnot. If you do not control your appetite, if you eat what you want and as much as you want, you can be sure of one thing: you will grow old fast and your physical personality will fall away fast too, or be completely wanting.

Overfeeding and wrong feeding will produce in the body a kind of self-poisoning (autointoxication) that can be as harmful as narcotics. Bright's disease, a degeneration of the kidneys that results in imperfect elimination of uric acid, usually is the result of an abused and constantly overloaded digestive tract. The enormous amount of poison that must be thrown off through the kidneys subjects them to overwork and impairment until they finally cannot function properly any longer.

You will be wise, before eating any food, to ask yourself some simple questions like these: Does this food contain the elements my body needs? And if so, how much of it do I need to eat? Don't eat because the food looks good or tastes good; be sure that it is good for you from a health standpoint.

Weak or strong, says Roland Ervin Howarth, you cannot fool nature. Sooner or later, violations of the laws of nature catch up with you. There is no good reason to fight nature, to ignore her rules of good nutrition, to deplete your health with modern foods that are devitalized, demineralized, roasted, toasted,

puffed, tenderized, artificially colored and flavored, and chemi-
calized with more than seven hundred potentially dangerous
chemical additives. The result will always be the same: sickness,
pain, suffering, and eventually death. E. G. White says:

> Many are made sick by indulgence of their appetite. They eat
> what suits their perverted taste, thus weakening the digestive
> organs, and injuring their power to assimilate the food that is to
> sustain life. Thus the delicate machinery is worn out by the
> suicidal practices of those who ought to know better. Sin indeed
> lies at the door, and the door is the mouth.
>
> If the appetite is allowed to rule, the mind will be brought
> under its control. The declension in virtue and the degeneracy of
> the race are chiefly attributable to the indulgence of perverted
> appetite.
>
> One of the strongest temptations that man has to meet is at the
> point of appetite. Christ began His work of redemption by
> reforming the physical habits of man.

Self-examination will bring the conviction home to you that
reform in your present living habits is imperative, and that many
of these habits must be changed if your body is to become a
charming graceful personality. Healthful living is the only road to
zest and vigor, vitality and longevity.

The character and size of this volume only allows a certain
amount of guidance and a few roadmarks to health reform. For a
fuller study of the subject, the health-food centers throughout the
country offer a good selection of books along this line. If what you
really want is an impressive personality, and longevity with
youthfulness and vigor, here are four books, all excellent, that you
should acquire, study diligently, and whose precepts you should
faithfully practice.* For the rest of your life you will be glad you
did so.

---

* *The Ministry of Healing*, E. G. White (Pacific Press, Mountain View,
Calif.); *Sally's Recipes for Better Nutrition*, S. D. Zerfing (P.O. Box 226,
Glendale, Calif.); *What's Missing in Your Body and Diet and Salad Suggestions*,
Dr. N. W. Walker, D.Sc. (Norwalk Press Publ., P.O. Box 13206, Phoenix,
Arizona).

There is great hope for those who tip the scale too heavily, who, as a result, have an unattractive appearance and suffer ill health, and who are unhappy with their physical personality. Remember, your body, in the final analysis, is merely the product of what you have eaten—past tense. Look into the looking glass. If you do not like what you see, and you want to change your physical appearance, just change your intake (out of which your body is made) and you will soon be pleased. There is much truth in the old saying: "What you eat today will walk and talk tomorrow."

Food plays a foremost role and is the all controlling and governing factor in your physical and mental development. On the selection, combination, and proportion of the food you ingest hinges your ability to reach the highest state of vitality, youthfulness, and perfect personality.

The first thing to do is to cut down on the amount of food you eat. Cut it in half, or, better, start a three-day fast. This will give nature a chance to do a cleaning job. You will feel much better, and build the expectancy of a longer life, if you reduce the quantity of your food intake.

In a later chapter we will show that food is not what you have to depend on for energy. Let me say now that you will not grow weak, rather you will gain in strength by cutting down on your food intake. This may seem paradoxical and contradictory, and not what you have hitherto believed. Nevertheless it is the truth.

Some years ago, Professor Huxley, of England, performed an interesting experiment with earthworms. He fed a whole family of earthworms, except one, the common way. To the one he gave the same food, but took it away for short periods, inserting fast days. This worm outlived nineteen generations of his brothers and sisters. For worm or man, the natural laws work in the same way.

By overeating, the excess food clogs the system, poisons the body, and may result in early death. By fasting at repeated intervals, the excess food and poison in the worm were eliminated, resulting in a longer life. Cut down on your eating; get rid of the poison; and you will feel better and live longer. This is the law of nature. It works that way for any living creature, be it worm, beast, or man.

Drink plenty of water. How much? There is no rule that can be applied to everyone. It will depend on what kind of food you eat, what kind of work you do, what kind of a constitution you have. Drink enough so that the body mechanism can do its cleansing work. Whether the cleansing is done through the pores of the skin, or through the lungs, kidneys, or bowels, fluid is needed to dissolve and expel toxins from the body.

What do you drink? Coffee, tea, coke, liquor, beer? All these drinks are toxins and of no help to the body in its cleansing work. We will consider these fluids later. They are all poisonous, harmful, and detrimental to the development of a perfect personality. Clean, fresh well water is good, but something the good Lord of Creation has prepared for us is still better, and nothing can exceed its value in cleansing, in building, and in maintaining our physical personality. Let Dr. N. W. Walker tell us the story of water:

> When we speak of water, the first thought is quite naturally of that which comes from the faucet, or from the spring, or even rain water. Few people stop to wonder if, or even realize that, there is vital organic as well as inorganic water.
>
> Water is composed of chemical elements, and the only way in which it can be organic, in other words, instilled with the life principle, is through the vegetable kingdom.
>
> The chemicals of the mineral kingdom are dead, and inorganic, but when dissolved by Nature and absorbed in plant life, or vegetation, then they become organicized with the life principle and so become organic.
>
> Nature has furnished vegetation as a laboratory in which to convert the inorganic water of rain and streams into life-containing atoms of vital organic water.
>
> The water from the faucet is not only inorganic, the atoms composing it being mineral elements entirely devoid of the life principle, but nearly all cities contaminate the water supply

with inorganic chlorine and other chemicals, making it truly unfit for human and animal consumption.

The destruction of life in fruits and vegetables by means of fire, excessive heat, or manufacturing processes, reconverts the organic chemicals back into their inorganic lifeless state.

This applies equally to water. Whether it comes from the faucet, from the spring, from rain, or is distilled, water is *inorganic.*

The only source from which vital organic water is derived is vegetation. The water when fed to vegetation is absorbed into the plant and becomes organic. Therefore, the raw juice from all fruits and vegetables is the finest organic water obtainable.

Be sure to study Dr. Walker's book on raw vegetable juices, referred to before. Live vegetable and fruit juices require no work on the part of the digestive apparatus, but are absorbed directly into the blood within fifteen minutes. They are the finest cleanser for obesity, and builder for physical personality.

Avoid milk and milk products. This is an incrimination of milk, and will come to some people quite unexpectedly, perhaps even as a shock. Immediately, the question will be raised: Is milk not one of the mainstays of our nutrition? Sorry, we cannot answer that question in the affirmative. A cow is a cow, and nature intended cow's milk for the little calf, not for humans. But we use cow's milk for ourselves, for our babies, for our children, and for our old folks. We use cow juice in our coffee, tea, cocoa, in sauces, in bread, in cake, in pudding, in ice cream, and what have you. We use cow's milk in the morning, at noon, in the evening, on Sundays, holidays, and weekdays, 365 days a year. Some housewives cannot cook, and some dieticians cannot make a menu, without cow juice.

Must a cow be the wet nurse for our babies, a source of fluid for our children, ourselves, and our senior citizens? If it is true that we are what we eat and drink, what conclusion shall we reach from these facts? Could it possibly be in the program of our Creator, when he said: "Let us make man in our image, after our likeness" (Gen. 1:26)?

We lived in China for nearly a quarter of a century. The Chinese do not drink milk, and wonder why foreigners want a cow as wet nurse for their babies, and cow's milk for their children and themselves. The Chinese have good body lines, few obesity cases, and hardly any body hair. I once overheard a discussion about why foreigners have so much body hair. The questioner was told by his friend that "cows have plenty of body hair, and cows are the wet nurses of the foreigners; what wonder then that they have so much body hair." Could it be that he had a point there?

In the last one hundred and fifty years, cow's milk has become a money-making business. It now belongs to the "Big Three," that is, the three biggest industries in the country, tobacco, alcohol, and milk. Milk is consumed in an amount that exceeds a billion gallons a year, extracted from more than 25,000,000 wet nurses, the cows. This is truly a gigantic business, isn't it? We now can understand the reason for the constant campaign on television: drink more milk for your health, feed more milk to your children for better development, and so on. But some may say: "My doctor tells me to drink more milk and prescribed more milk for my baby and my children." Of course, not all doctors do this. There are many doctors who neither ride the milk-wagon train, cherish the cocktail lunch, nor patronize the tobacco syndicate.

In this study let us make it clear: milk is one of the culprits, if not the main one, responsible in the case of 41,000,000 Americans who suffer from obesity and the deformation of their physical personality. This is a fact. Therefore, let us have the arraignment and the answer to the indictment right now.

What is milk? Milk is a sex product, a secretion from the mammary glands of female mammals and women. The Creator designed the mammary glands and their secretion for the nourishment of offspring immediately after their birth. It was designed as a temporary measure, just for the weaning period. When the young grow enough teeth to eat stronger food, milk drinking or sucking is discontinued. This law is observed throughout the mammal world; only humans are guilty of its violation.

The Creator further designed for each species a fixed composition of its milk, just right for its use. For instance, a calf weighs perhaps forty pounds at birth, a human baby usually not more than ten pounds, or less. A calf can walk the very first day it is born; therefore the Creator, in His infinite wisdom, designed cow's milk to contain four times as much calcium and four times as much protein as human milk.

In nature, each species weans its own offspring. Only humans are guilty of violating this procedure; they get a cow to wean their babies. But the Creator ruled: "Let the earth bring forth the living creature after his kind, cattle . . . after his kind, and it was so" (Gen. 1:24). Furthermore, the Creator designed things so that the juice of the mammary glands should not come in contact with contaminated air or destructive light by creating teats. From the teats the milk should thus pass directly from the mother into the stomach of the offspring. This rule also is observed by the mammal world; only humans are guilty of its violation. They artificially extract the juice from the mammary glands of the cow, in violation of the natural law.

Dr. A. J. Goodfellow, a British physician, has this to say about the violation of this natural law:

> When nature forms the milk in the mammary glands it is sterile, and her intention is that it should pass directly from the gland through the teats straight into the stomach of the offspring without contaminating air or destructive action of light. When we frustrate, defy or disregard any of nature's laws—nature usually exacts the appropriate penalty. The trouble is that the punishment may come such a long time after the crime that we fail to link up the two in the relationship of cause and effect, and thus fail to profit by experience.
>
> Consider, for example, the millions of young lives that have been sacrificed in the last century through our persistent disregard of nature's intention. All the deaths that have occurred through drinking contaminated milk, all the epidemics that have occurred from milk-borne infections. A great many of these cases

should never have occurred if we would have kept our milk from contact with air and light.

The doctor closes with the old proverb: "The mills of the Lord grind very slow, but they grind exceeding fine."

Is this not true? The United States, the nation that consumes the greatest amount of milk and milk products, has become the leading country of the world in the number of its people afflicted with degenerative diseases.

Dr. Frank J. Wilson, D.O., discusses the subject as follows:

> Among the nations of the world, the United States is a leader in the material things it has provided for its people. But it is also a leader in some of the least desirable things, such as degenerative diseases. We think of our national nutrition as reaching higher and higher levels, but at the same time records show steady inroads from diseases such as hardening of the arteries, degenerative heart diseases, hypertension with heart disease, rheumatism, arthritis, diabetes mellitus, cancer, and a host of other degenerative afflictions, including unabated growth in dental difficulties.

Then he asks this sensible question: "Can we, at the same time, be a nation with improved nutrition, and increasing degenerative disorders? Facts and common sense deny such a theory." Dr. Michael Rabben, D.D.S., asks this question:

> If milk, cow's milk, that is, is so good nutritionally, why has it not done all the good expected of it? It is well known that children drinking lots of cow's milk still have a great deal of tooth decay. Pediatricians also confirm the fact that heavy milk drinkers have anemia, allergies, asthma, rickets, excessive lymph-oid, proliferation, endocrine malfunction such as hypogonadism, and even possibly cancer, through overstimulation of the anterior pituitary.

"Once a child is weaned, milk is never afterwards a suitable food," asserts Dr. F. M. Collins.

The Creator designed milk as a food for the newborn. And it is a perfect food, since it is similar to the blood in its composition. The Chinese do not drink milk; they call it bae hsueh, which means white blood, and they think that the white man's custom of drinking "white blood" is a survival of his former barbarism.

Dr. J. A. Goodfellow makes this contribution:

> For all practical purpose milk may be regarded as "blood" minus its red coloring matter. The red blood corpuscles are no longer required to carry oxygen, because the offspring is now able to produce its own oxygen from its lungs by means of its own red blood cells.—In all other respects the composition of milk resembles the composition of blood.

It seems that the Chinese have a true point in their conception of "white blood." The Creator designed this life-giving, perfect food to pass from mother to offspring in a direct way, by way of the teats. In His infinite wisdom, God made special provision for the digestion of the milk in the stomach of the newborn. He provided a glandular layer that secretes an enzyme known as rennin, or chymosin, which curdles, ferments, and digests the milk. And the marvelous thing is that this enzyme production stops when the weaning period ends. Adults lack rennin, or chymosin, and have no enzyme production for the digestion of milk. This is the way nature lets us know that milk is a food for babies, and babies only.

This is also why the human body, after being weaned, no longer has the ability, except in very rare cases, to utilize milk of animal origin as constructive nourishment. Further, for children and adults, milk is the most mucus-forming food we have. This can be readily understood when we realize that the quantity of casein in cow's milk is more than 300 per cent greater than that in human milk, and since the secretion of rennin has been stopped by divine decree in children and adults, there are no enzymes to break up and digest the casein.

The best glue a cabinetmaker can use to fasten wooden boards together is made from the casein in cow's milk. What happens to the indigestible casein in the chronic violator of the natural law, the chronic milk drinker and eater of cow's milk products? It becomes the stuff the cabinetmaker uses—glue. And this glue that accumulates from the daily intake of milk and milk products clogs up the whole human system, and is often the real cause of the so-called common colds, which is nature's effort to get rid of the accumulated mucus glue in the system.

It has long been thought that germs are the factor that causes the common cold, but no one has ever isolated them. Could not this be the real cause of the common cold and the answer to why research workers cannot find any "germ"?

Dr. M. K. Yergin states:

> It is a widely demonstrated fact among physicians of careful observation in the effect of varied articles of diet, that milk uniformly causes a clogged condition of the human system.

And Dr. Walker adds:

> There is no cure for colds so long as milk is used—whereas, children who have been trained not to drink milk nor to eat milk products are usually immune to this affliction.

Julius Gilbert White, in Abundant Health, states:

> The highest degree of immunity to colds is secured by using the strict vegetarian ration, without the use of milk, cream, cottage cheese, butter and eggs.

God is no respecter of persons, and here is what He says about milk and the users of milk: "Newborn babes desire milk" (I Pet. 2:2); "Every one that useth milk is unskilful . . . for he is a babe" (Heb. 5:13); and "Strong food belongs to them that are of full age" (Heb. 5:14). And He promises to teach knowledge to "them who are weaned from the milk" (Isa. 28:9).

In answer to the first question, What is milk? we have found that it is baby food only, and a baby food from the mother directly to her offspring.

Correctly, human mother's milk to the human baby, and cow's milk from the mother cow to the calf.

OBESITY, MILK AND GROWTH

In obesity we deal with a phenomenon that is common to at least every fifth American (there are about 41,000,000 victims) and a dangerous hazard to the rest of the nation. An insurance survey has disclosed the startling fact that the mortality rate for those who are ten to twenty pounds overweight is 94 per cent above normal, whatever that is, and for those who are fifty pounds overweight it is 153 per cent above the normal. This should be enough evidence to show that obesity carries with it a sure promise of an earlier grave than is necessary. Everyone who is not so afflicted should meditate earnestly this phrase, "This can happen to me," and then try to understand the situation and take appropriate steps to avoid the calamity. Professor Engles contends that "we understand a phenomenon only if we examine its origin and genealogy." If this is so, we have no right to be dogmatic, intolerant, or prejudiced against a truth that may appear. We must examine without bias each phenomenon, each experience, each natural law, even if it should reveal the truth of a matter to be contrary to conventional belief and practice.

There is more than one cause for obesity, but in my considered opinion the main cause, besides starch and sweets, will be found in the milk diet. According to recent figures from the United States Department of Agriculture, "The average yearly consumption of milk and milk products amounts to approximately 418 lbs. per person, child and adult."

The proportion is greater during infancy and childhood, when we lay the foundation for future health or ill health. We would be wise, therefore, to protect our nation's health by looking into the milk problem. In my sojourn among the people of the Far East I observed very closely their mode of living, their figures and body contours, and I am thoroughly convinced of this: The more than a billion people of the Far East—China, Japan, India, Malaysia—do not live on a milk diet and do not indulge in milk drinking after the weaning period. In this respect they live more in conformity with the laws of nature, and the terrific contrast in fine bone structure and body lines in their favor forcefully drives home the truth.

Obesity is called a degenerative disease; modified, we will say, it is the base of many degenerative diseases enumerated before. To degenerate means to decline, to deteriorate, to become inferior. Since the drinking of cow's milk is acclaimed by so many, even by a great part of the medical profession, as good and healthful, how then can such a wide area of bad health be blamed on it? Evidence should give clearer understanding, and furnish an answer to the how and why.

After the weaning period, what are the effects of a milk diet on the physical and mental structures of a personality?

Answer: The overdevelopment of the skeletal structure of the body, a fattening of the constitution, and the distortion of normal body lines. The under development of the nervous structure and a lowering of the mentality.

For the development and maintenance of the physical and mental qualities, a person largely depends on the internal secretions. Whether he is to be tall or short, fat or slender, depends mainly upon the proper function of the endocrine system and particularly upon the secretion and hormones of the pituitary gland.

What is the endocrine system, and what are glands and hormones? What are their functions in the process of developing a personality?

Answer: They are the main and mysterious factors in our physical as well as in our intellectual building program. So let us get acquainted with them.

THE ENDOCRINE SYSTEM: GLANDS

Glands are bodily organs designed by the Creator to secrete special fluids and material essential for the development and the maintenance of our physical and mental personality. Normal functions and activities of the glands are the absolute basis for a normal personality. Underactivity or overactivity of the glands can produce an abnormal personality. Obesity, everyone will agree, is an abnormality, and its cause may be found in the activities of the glands. The glands are divided into two classes: the exocrine, or duct glands, and the endocrine, or ductless glands. Though the exocrine glands are important to bodily function, the most important in personality building are the endocrine, or ductless, glands.

Let us name the most important, starting at the top of the frame, and following down the line as follows: the pineal, the pituitary, the thyroid, the thymus, the adrenals, the pancreas, the prostate, and the gonads (testicles and ovaries).

These endocrine glands work together as a team. Collectively, they are known as the endocrine system. They are complementary to each other and are involved in every function of the human economy. They produce and discharge directly into the blood or lymph stream the so-called true hormones, and play a very prominent role in developing and maintaining our body system. They are of immense significance to our state of well-being, and what we really are, physically and mentally, largely depends on them. Growth, weight, stature of the body, structure of skin and hair, our voice and tone, our emotions and excitements, our whole being—all are influenced and controlled by the hormones of the endocrine system. The study of them is indeed interesting and highly fascinating.

Dr. Barker declares:

> More and more we are forced to realize that the general form and external appearance of the human body depends to a large extent upon the functioning of the endocrine glands. Our stature, the kind of face we have, the length of our arms and legs, the shape of the pelvis, the color and consistency of our skin, the quantity and regional location of our fat, the amount and distribution of hair on our bodies, the tonicity of our muscles, the sound of our voice, and the size of the larynx, the emotions to which our exterior gives expression, all are, to a certain extent, conditioned by the production of our endocrine glands. We are, in a sense, the beneficiaries or victims of the chemical correlations of our endocrine organs, and their hormones.

THE   ENDOCRINE   SYSTEM: HORMONES

The word hormones comes from the Greek *hormaein*, which means to set in motion, to excite. It is a chemical substance produced by the glands and carried by the blood or lymph stream to another part of the system, on which it has a stimulating, exciting effect, increasing functional activity.

Dr. A. I. Brown has this to say about the hormones:

Some hormones increase the rapidity of your heart action; others slow it down. Some raise blood pressure; others lower it. The rate of your breathing, the pace of your digestive processes, the clearness of your vision, the strength of your bones, the alertness of your brain, the nature of your disposition are all affected by the hormones.

There is some resemblance to those drugs taken in with food. These are called vitamins. If vitamin A is missing, your eyes go bad; if vitamin B is absent or reduced, your nerves go bad; if vitamin C is not sufficient, the dentist will get you; if vitamin D is less than normal, bone troubles are likely.

But, compared to the hormones of the ductless glands, vitamins seem very commonplace. Some endocrine hormones seem so powerful that one thirty-thousandth of a grain is an effective dose. And these small doses are necessary to life, although a much larger amount would kill speedily.

Hormones may be called the officers of the human system. They command, direct, set things in motion, get things done, but they do not do the work themselves. They are very enthusiastic about their work; they excite.

Here is an illustration. An insemination has occurred in the ovaries, and immediately the pituitary gland goes into action and releases an army of prolactin hormones, which stimulate lactation, and antuitrin, the growth hormones, into the bloodstream. They travel quickly and directly to the mammary glands, exciting them to action, to get ready and produce milk, the life food for the offspring. And as the hormones order and excite, the mammary glands obey and provide, and when the offspring is born the food it needs is ready and waiting. Indeed, with the psalmist we may exclaim: "We praise thee, O Lord; we are fearfully and wonderfully made" (Ps. 139:14).

THE PITUITARY GLAND

The pituitary gland is known as the master gland, the controller, the co-ordinator of the whole endocrine system. It now is generally believed that all the glands of the system are under the control and direction of the pituitary.

Next to the pineal gland, the pituitary is located on the highest level in the human economy, right on the under surface of the brain just behind the nasal cavities, and adjoining the thalamus in the sella turcica, or Turk's saddle. It is a small reddish-gray body, the size of a large pea, about one centimeter in diameter and weighs only 6 to 10 grains. It consists of a tuberal part and two lobes, anterior and posterior, or front and back lobes, each manufacturing its own specific hormones. It is believed that one manufactures hormones for the feminine and the other for the masculine characteristics. The work that the Creator has allotted this mysterious little gland is amazingly great and unbelievably diversified; it is the most interesting chemical and drug factory known to exist in the human economy. Eleven distinct hormones are known, four in the posterior lobe, and seven in the anterior lobe. But medical researchers believe there are, and they are looking for, many more. The gland's scope of activity is so wide that it has not yet been definitely established. Let us just name a few of these activities: blood-pressure control, blood-supply control, salt-content control, body-temperature control, body-growth control, body-fluid control, some phases of metabolism, especially phosphorus metabolism, sex control, appetite control, emotional control, and whatnot. It seems that nothing goes on in the human body over which the pituitary gland does not have control.

The pituitary, through its hormone activities, definitely controls the two major life forces, reproduction and growth. And here lies the greatest interest in our study of the phenomenon of obesity and its cause and genealogy, which we concluded might be found in the American milk diet.

> 1. For reproduction, the pituitary produces the gonadotropic hormones, prolan A, and prolan B, by which the gonads, testicles, and ovaries are stimulated and excited to produce other necessary hormones for reproduction.
>
> 2. For growth, the pituitary produces the prolactin hormones, which excite the mammary glands to milk production, and antuitrin G, which excites the bones and skeletal frame to expand and enlarge.

Milk is a sexual fluid, loaded with all these hormones and other growth material. It is the medium of nourishment for the offspring from the time of birth until it is transferred from the mother supply to another form of nourishment. The offspring needs these hormones from the mother's pituitary and sex glands for its first year's growth, which is the most rapid growth in its life. This is true of a human babe as well as all mammals.

Dr. Walker says:

> Each milk fed species of animals generates the kind and quality of milk best suited for the structure of the skeleton and the rest of the frame of the body of its own species. Such milk is intended for nourishment *only* from the birth up to the age of weaning.

Weaning periods are of different duration for each species: for humans, 18 to 20 months; for calves, 6 to 8 months; for lambs, 4 to 5 months; for pigs, 2 months; and so on. Weaning, according to Webster's Dictionary, means "to accustom a child or young animal to take nourishment otherwise than by nursing." And according to the *Encyclopaedia Britannica*, "to transfer the young from the dependency on its mother's milk to another form of nourishment."

The Bible speaks of milk, but to the best of my knowledge it does not mention specifically the milk of the cow, not even once. The cow's milk we drink contains plenty of growth and sex hormones from the cow's pituitary. But these are not healthy hormones, either; in fact, they are sickly and feverish, produced by an unnatural overstimulation of the cow's endocrine glandular system, and have a detrimental effect in the human body.

The plain truth is set down by J. I. Rodale in *Prevention*. He writes:

> Man has made a milk factory, a machine, out of the cow. Normally the cow gave about 200 lbs. of milk in a year to wean her calf. Today there are cows that give 15,000 lbs. of milk, or 75 times as much. And this overproduction is causing more diseases in cows; many have leukemia, others tuberculosis a.s.o. When we force a cow to give 75 times the amount of milk God had intended her to give, it must be milk that is not up to snuff. That is point one. And point two is "artificial insemination." The dairymen seem to delight in making a cow a complete artificial animal. Formerly a bull mated with a cow in order to give her a calf, but that is too much trouble for dairymen today, so they have this artificial insemination. The bull is masturbated and the amount of semen ejaculated is used to inject into forty or fifty cows, or even more. It is nothing more than male prostitution. It is an irreligious, impious trick if I ever saw one. First they hang a hundred pound weight under the cow, then they deprive her of her gentleman friend. What next? They are piling artificiality upon artificiality. Poor bossy, with her sad eyes, waiting for the father of her children who never comes. One day she may realize that she has been let down, deceived, tricked, cheated out of the natural biological satisfaction which is her inherent right. Can the milk of such a cow be any good?

Here is an answer to that question by Dr. Frank J. Wilson, one of America's leading endocrinologists. He says:

> Normally a cow produced about two to four quarts of milk a day. But through selective breeding, a dairy cow now has a capacity of several gallons of milk daily. How was this accomplished? By breeding what some authorities call "endocrine freaks" or *cows with overactive anterior pituitary glands* which naturally produce excessive quantities of the anterior pituitary hormone along with the milk. What this higher quantity of pituitary hor-

mone does to the human system is easily detected (obesity, over-sized bone structures), especially in the younger generation, which is developing physical characteristics that should be viewed with concern rather than pride.

Here is one of many cases:

The father of a seventeen year old boy came to me when he was concerned about the boy's abnormal size, and lack of youthful energy. I learned from the father that the boy was a habitually heavy milk drinker, sometimes more than two quarts a day. The boy should not weigh 285 lbs., and be six feet five inches in height. Instead of having a normal boy's enthusiasm, he was sluggish and lacked stamina. When I examined him I noted a widening of the pelvis, with broadening hips. And, of course, he had far too much fat on his body. In his case the development of the skeletal system had outrun development of the nervous and glandular systems. As a result, the body cannot make uniform progress. As more milk hormones are taken into the body, they produce more growth, but the principle question is whether some types of growth are desirable.

There is strong evidence that the hormonal constituent of milk may be the factor in constant growing metabolic problems and in altered growth characteristics, detrimental to health and normal body development and function.

The success in a reducing diet requires that all growth-stimulating factors be removed. Since milk is so high in growth elements, I insist that milk be eliminated from the diet of those I treat for weight reduction.

Artificial milk production is possible only by overstimulating the cow's pituitary, and thus the milk we drink is overloaded with gonadotropic, prolactin, antuitrin, and other cow hormones. The more we drink of this milk, the more of these feverish cow hormones we take into our system. In turn, these hormones over-stimulate our own pituitary-growth hormones, and the result is overdevelopment of our bone structure and a fattening of the constitution. The victim becomes slow, dull, and sleepy, in different degrees, and we have before us the phenomenon of obesity. And with it goes more often than not the underdevelopment of the nerve structure, and a lowering of the mentality. Dr. M. K. Yergin, concludes:

You do not know what it is to be in perfect condition as a full grown [human being] on a milk diet. I advise you to test it out for yourself and know the truth.

Dr. P. H. Goddard, of Ohio State University, made this statement:

Seventy per cent of the adults of the United States haven't the intelligence of an average ten year old student, and a change in the school system is necessary.

Dr. James A. Goodfellow adds this:

The number of mental defectives and backward children is increasing at an alarming rate. And it will go on increasing. Most children do not have sufficient brain power to absorb enough education in eight years to fit them for life, so the school-leaving age had to be raised to fifteen, then sixteen, seventeen, and finally to eighteen. Will eighteen be enough? Professor Dors Moran made this statement: "Most of the young men, none under eighteen, who have chosen the medical profession as a career, are incapable of accurate observation, unable to reason correctly from observed facts, and generally are deficient in intelligence. As a class they are unfit to make satisfactory doctors.

Here is another statement by Dr. M. K. Yergin:

Education is not what makes intelligence. Education can train intelligence, but when intelligence is deficient there is always a lack of those energies which characterize human beings as the image of God. It is a widely demonstrated fact among physicians of careful observation in the effect of varied articles of diet that milk uniformly causes two definite conditions within the human being: (1) lowered mentality, and (2) a clogged condition of the system.

Nature designed cow's milk, for the nourishment of a baby cow. A baby cow's intelligence is never very high at its best. And a full-grown cow has scarcely a degree of intelligence, any intelligent capacity to be coveted by normal human beings.

Cow's milk has not in it the elements and material for the development of anything but cow's intelligence, and this is in the infant stage. Is it then to be wondered that the widespread milk habit of Americans has reduced the mentality of 70% of American adults to that of a boy ten years of age?

Dr. Frank J. Wilson says:

Among mammals, cows are in the lower range of the scale where the nervous system and the brain are concerned. So it is not surprising that the ratio of elements required for the nourishment of a calf is not the same as the ratio of elements needed by a child. This fact is borne out in milk studies.

Do you think you are paying your child a compliment, when you feed it a fluid nature intended for the nourishment of a baby beast? Is the human child with its marvelous brain, mind and soul not worthy of the very best? Is it not worth more than the juice of a mentally inferior beast? This appeals to the common sense.

Human milk is for human babies, and when a substitute is necessary there is available soya milk and almond milk, both of which are very nourishing and do not clog the human system. They are not the same as mother's milk, but much better than cow's milk, and they are good for every age.

As for adults, avoid cow's milk. God our Creator gave us the highest parts of herbs, their seeds, and the fruit of the trees for our food. Fruit and vegetable juices develop the highest type of intelligence, make the best base for spirituality, prolong youthfulness indefinitely, and assure longevity. Under such a natural program, obesity, in most cases, will disappear, and graceful body lines for a charming physical personality will be developed.

Soybean milk in liquid or powder form as marketed today is simple, delicious, and very palatable. Personally, we use the Loma Linda Food Company's product, and Soyalac or Soyamel, put out by the Worthington Food Company.

For infants and children, the Loma Linda Food Company manufactures a special-brand "hypoallergenic" powder to use as milk.

MILK ANALYSIS

(United States Department of Agriculture,
Bureau of Chemistry and Soil, Washington D.C.)

MILK	WATER	ASH	PROTEIN	FAT	CARBOHYDRATES
Human milk	89.95%	0.25%	1.30%	2.50%	6.00%
Soybean milk	87.03%	0.52%	2.40%	3.15%	6.90%
Nut milk	87.00%	2.03%	5.60%	5.60%	7.23%
Cow's milk	87.30%	0.80%	3.20%	3.20%	5.20%
Goat's milk	87.00%	0.50%	4.00%	4.50%	4.00%

Soybean milk *does not contain cholesterol*, a fatty monatomic crystalline alcohol found in meat and some animal products. It is an important component in forming gallstones and in hardening of the arteries.

Soybean milk is *free of streptococci*, a bacteria that includes a highly pathogenic species that causes many diseases, such as pneumonia, erysipelas, and others. (Professor George W. Cav-anaugh, professor of chemistry at Cornell University, who is quoted by D. C. Jarvis, M.D., in *Arthritis and Folk Medicine*, has this to say about cow's milk: "You have streptococci in the milk [cow's milk] at any time you care to feed the cow a high protein diet. Dairymen depend on high protein feed to speed up the milk and butterfat production.")

Soybean milk can be easily digested. It does not form hard curds in the stomach. It does not putrefy as cow's milk or goat's milk does. It is a vegetable product and does not require the enzyme rennin, so necessary for human and animal milk digestion.

Soybean milk will clabber, and can be made into cheese that is easy to digest. In China, they call soybean milk *tou yang*, and the cheese *tou fu*, which we enjoyed very much.

Soybean milk and its products are highly alkaline and well adapted for the human system, both for children and adults. Soybean milk is infinitely better for human consumption than

cow's milk or goat's milk. It is not contaminated by animal contact; it is free of disease germs; and is not liable to putrefy.

Soybean milk is a laxative, whereas cow's milk may cause
constipation. (Professor J. G. White, in Abundant Health, asks: "If
soybean milk makes sick babies well, would it be good for babies
who are now well? Would it not help to protect them from future
illness?")

The soybean is the best protein food with which America is
blessed. It is also called "the wonder food of the world."

11. ALCOHOL AND PERSONALITY

ALCOHOL AND personality do not fit together.

Here are the cold, factual findings of a Los Angeles grand jury,
as reported in *The Christum Century*: "Our jails and prisons are
crowded. Our courts and police organizations are burdened; our
law enforcement and social welfare are seriously aggravated
because of the licensed liquor traffic. The tax costs now falling to
the innocent citizenry, because of the liquor traffic, are intol-
erable."

The amount spent annually for liquor in the United States is the
unbelievable sum of nine billion dollars. In addition a good part of
the twelve to fifteen billion dollars per year spent for police, jails,
courts, and hospitals is connected with cases involving alcohol.
Besides this, Uncle Sam is cheated out of a large share of the
excise tax for twenty per cent of all alcohol (about 61,000,000
gallons), or every fifth bottle, consumed in 1960 was bootlegged.

If America could only be sober and abstain from alcohol for
three years, the money saved could pay all its debts, and the tax
burden of its citizens could be reduced by more than 50 per cent.
In developing a program of personality building, we must

urge the avoidance of alcohol in any amount, at any time. But this seems as hard a problem to solve as the avoidance of milk for one's nutritional good.

Today, millions of people believe that a social drink is a part of modern life and congenial society. They feel a loftiness when participating in, or giving, cocktail parties. Here is what Ann Landers, a noted columnist, says:

> Most women who say they must take a drink to be sociable are only kidding themselves. You will have to go a long way to find one who is more sociable than I am. Yet, I have never needed liquor as a crutch.
>
> When I attend cocktail parties, as I often do, I merely say: "Ginger ale, please!" and I am not a bit uncomfortable. A woman who is able to say no, so that it sounds like no and not maybe should have no problem.

Many comfort themselves with the belief that they only participate in moderate drinking. While no one can seriously maintain that the excessive use of alcohol, or the condition of intoxication, is harmless and desirable, a great many people do believe and maintain that the "moderate" use of alcohol is harmless. The fact is, however, that "moderate drinking" is the school in which people are educated and from which they are graduated for a drunkard's career. There is not a drunkard in the world, and there never has been one, who has not started in the school of moderate drinking. So insidious is this education that the highway of drunkenness is entered before the victim suspects the danger.

Dr. Andrew C. Ivy, the famous authority on drinking and alcohol problems, says this:

> Most delinquency, broken homes and felonies are either directly or indirectly the result of drinking, which costs the American taxpayer from 50 to 60 billion dollars every year. It is estimated that for every dollar spent for alcoholic beverages, five dollars are needed to repair the damages. Alcohol in even small amounts increases the accident rate, killing and maiming thousands all over the country.

There is no getting away from it, alcohol is a habit-forming drug and causes mental, moral and physical deterioration. It brings misery and suffering to the wife and children of the victim. There is no harmless alcoholic beverage. Beer, wine, rum, gin, whisky, all of these contain alcohol.

The habit of drinking intoxicating liquors is a great evil, and no moral character can have any part in it. From the powerful pen of E. G. White, we have the following narration:

> Every year millions upon millions of gallons of intoxicating liquors are consumed. Millions upon millions of dollars are spent in buying *wretchedness, poverty, disease, degeneration, lust, crime,* and *death.* For the sake of gain, the liquor-seller deals out to his victims that which corrupts and destroys mind and body. He entails on the drunkard's family poverty and wretchedness.
>
> There is no class guilty of greater perversion and abuse of God's precious gifts than those who employ the products of the soil in the manufacture of intoxicating liquors. The nutritive grains, the healthful, delicious fruits are converted into beverages that *pervert the sense and madden the brain.* As a result of the use of these poisons, thousands of families are deprived of the comfort and even the necessities of life. Acts of violence and crimes are multiplied, and disease and death hurry myriads of victims to a drunkard's grave.
>
> This work of destruction is carried on under the protection of the law of the land. For a paltry sum men are licensed to deal out to their fellow men the potion that shall rob them of all hope of the life to come. Our laws sustain an evil which is sapping their very foundation.

Criminal courts and prisons, almshouses, insane asylums and hospitals are all filled, to a great degree, as a result of liquor-selling. Day by day, month by month, year by year, this trade goes on. Fathers, husbands, brothers, the hope and pride of the nation, are steadily entering the liquor dealer's haunts, to be sent back wrecked and ruined.

More terrible yet, the course is striking at the very heart of the home. It is sad to say, but more and more, women are forming the liquor habit. Little children, even in the innocence and helplessness of babyhood, are in daily peril through the neglect, the abuse, and the vileness of drunken mothers.

Sons and daughters are growing up under the shadow of this terrible evil. What outlook do they have for their future? Nothing, except the possibility that they may sink even lower than their parents.

F.B.I. Director J. Edgar Hoover asserts:

> The startling increase in juvenile delinquency is largely due to parental failure. The drinking woman today probably deserves more than her statistical share of the blame for juvenile delinquency.

Alcohol is not only one of Western civilization's greatest problems, it is also one of its greatest curses. Pertinent facts are on record about the effects of alcohol on morality, mortality, and longevity. Here is a typical human-interest story as related by Evelyn Scott, in *Shadow Across the Afternoon*:

> When I am alone I seldom turn on the radio. The early morning news, the "Upward Look," and possibly the "Trading Post" are enough for me. I am not much for radio. But when the teenagers are home, it blares constantly. Over and over a fellow extols some brand of beer as "one of the finer things of life." I wonder!
>
> For I remember an August afternoon in Vanadium, New Mexico, not long ago, a beautiful afternoon, bright with sunlight and sweet with the scent of roses. I dug a flower bed under an ancient, shady oak tree, and the babies were deep in their afternoon sleep.
>
> A little farther up the canyon, at Hanover, a young miner left his home to go to Bayart. He was the kind of fellow you like to have for a neighbor, friendly, devoted to his family, a steady worker, never drunk, never in trouble.
>
> But today he did an unprecedented thing. He stopped at a bar, bought a can of beer and drank it as he drove along (to try out the radio advertising).
>
> This can of beer took the fine edge off his alertness. The mountain road was narrow, cut in the side of the hill. Presently he was driving a little out from the hill, a little on the wrong side, down the grade and up the hill. He met a huge Santa Fe

truck, head on. There was the sound of the crash, then nothing—nothing at all.

The little green coupe was crumpled, as a man might crumple a match box in his hand. The truck driver climbed down from his cab, his face ashen.

He struggled to open the jammed door. It would not budge. In a frenzy of haste he ran back to the truck, got an iron bar, and tried to pry open the door. Quite suddenly it did open. He dropped the iron bar to the ground and reached in, lifting the driver with infinite care.

There had not been any need to hurry, any need to be careful. The driver was past all hurrying and beyond all hurt. His slight form was heavy in the truck driver's arms. A thin trickle of blood flowed from a cut on the side of the face, marking a damp spot on the ground, but the heartbeat the truck driver strained so hard to hear was not there.

To have looked into that still young face, so remote in its calm, one might have thought he only slept and would presently waken. But a shadow lay across the bright afternoon—*the shadow of death.* There was no way to change it, no way to go back a few minutes and make it not so.

In the little green coupe, a beer can rested on the floor, its mission done!

"One of the finer things of life!" as advertised.

It is generally conceded by the proponents as well as by the opponents of alcohol that the typical drunkard will fill an early grave. But records and statistics show that unnumbered "occasional drinkers/' moderate drinkers, and nondrinkers fill early graves too, because of the result of alcohol.

In the foregoing story, only one can of beer brought the young man to death row, robbing his wife and children of a loving and caring husband and father. Not a drunkard, no, not even a moderate drinker, only an occasional drinker. A test would have shown an alcohol content in the blood of less than 0.05 per cent or one part alcohol in 2,000 parts of blood. The law would have passed him as sober, but not nature. Hear her voice saying: "One can of beer only is one can of beer too much" Too much to let the nervous system maintain its normal working order, and enough to send the violator to death row. And that is what happened.

How much do you know about the effects of alcohol? The law allows 0.15 per cent of alcohol in the blood. Why? Nobody knows. Perhaps in deference to the liquor industry? There is no logical or normal reason for such a law, because less than 0.15 per cent, even one per cent, is enough to affect the subject's mood, thoughts, self-control, and responsibility, as we saw in the foregoing story.

Several university laboratory psychologists have conducted scientifically controlled tests that definitely prove that even after one drink people do not function normally. The tests have shown that visual reaction is impaired 333 per cent, the ability to memorize poetry is impaired 50 per cent, the ability to solve mathematical problems is impaired 13 per cent, the ability to reason is impaired 67 per cent, and muscular strength is decreased 10 per cent. All this after just one drink. Avoid it! Consider these findings, especially if you are a student.

"It is estimated that a driver on the average has to cope with at least a hundred driving situations every mile on the highway. In the city it jumps to three hundred decisions. A nondrinking driver will make one wrong decision in every forty. A drinker will make at least 23 per cent more errors than the nondrinker." (*Cosmopolitan.*)

Alcohol requires no digestive processing. Like water, honey, and simple sugar glucose, it passes directly into the blood without any change. Its rate of assimilation depends on how much food is in the stomach and upper intestinal tract at the time of drinking. If the organs are practically empty, the alcohol is absorbed instantly into the blood stream and the system. The heart pumps the blood three times through the whole body within one minute, and blood tests taken only five minutes after drinking are positive. Alcohol is extremely diffusible, and passes with ease through all human membranes. Therefore the amount of alcohol found in the blood does *not* represent the fullness of the alcohol that has been absorbed. *It passes from the alimentary canal into the blood stream and likewise into all the tissues of the body, the brain included.* Therefore, if we find 0.05 per cent alcohol in the blood stream, we know that every body cell and every brain cell is saturated with the same amount. Furthermore, the brain cells of the central nervous system are very susceptible and readily affected by the paralyzing action of alcohol. This is why one who drinks even one can of beer, or one glass of liquor, partly loses control over his actions, and should not be trusted at the wheel of an automobile or with any heavy responsibility. An additional glass of liquor or an additional bottle of beer increases the amount of alcohol in the blood and tissues, and with it the paralytic effect on the brain cells, until, reaching the amount of 0.15 per cent or more, the alcohol content in the blood and the system effects a nearly complete loss of voluntary motion. Often, too, the ability to perceive sensations, and to talk and walk, is lost, and the victim ends in the gutter, a place for swine but not for human beings.

Here is a description of the effects of alcohol by two experts, Drs. E. M. Abrahamson and A. W. Pezet:

> The drinks that follow the first drink, one or two or three, steadily increase the concentration of alcohol in the blood. The anesthetizing effect moves from one region of the brain to another. After the highest centers have been dulled, and our judgment destroyed gradually but inexorably, the regions of muscular coordination, speech, and vision are affected. We begin to weave as we walk. We miss the end of the cigarette as we try to light it. Our speech becomes thick and slurred; our vision is blurred and eventually doubled. Sooner or later, as the higher faculties that make us human are all put to sleep, we become animals. [Not personalities!]

According to Dr. C. W. Muehlberger, Michigan State University toxicologist, ethyl alcohol, because of its wide use in social drinking, is at the top of the list of all poisons in seriousness of consequences. Although it does not directly cause as many deaths as carbon monoxide, its indirect toll in dead, permanently disabled, and seriously injured is far greater. Tests show that there is a measurable impairment of ability after a person drinks only one glass of beer or one ounce of whisky. The higher intellectual levels of the brain, which are the most essential in man's progress toward becoming a profitable human being, a personality able to make a free choice and control his destiny, are affected. The alcohol drinker may first feel exhilarated, a kind of loftiness. What is the true cause of this? It is caused by the action of the pituitary gland and the endocrine system. The pituitary, called by some the subconscious mind, is always on the alert. As soon as alcohol enters the body, it sends out an alarm to the whole system. The invader must be expelled!

What happens then? All the glands, especially the adrenals, send out hormones. These mysterious messengers to all the cells involved fight with the invading poison. The result is a feeling of exhilaration. But then the drinker takes another drink, the system becomes overloaded with the poison, and the faithful endocrine forces are overwhelmed, the exhilaration ends, and exhaustion is the result.

To make a fanciful comparison, one might say that drinking alcoholic beverages is like entering a time machine, in which the clock moves backward. In drinking liquor, *the process takes only a very short time to erase the highly developed functions of discrimination, judgment, and social consciousness, and lowers man to the level of the animals.*

Do we state too much if we say: "Drinking is degrading; its practice is unworthy of a personality?" If you strive to build up your personality, have the courage to say: "No thank you, I do not drink," and mean it.

Chaplain John E. Keplinger, U.S. Army, in interviewing Captain Clifford E. Keys, Jr., a famous non-drinking paratrooper who had 133 parachute jumps to his credit, asked: "What's the reason that you don't drink, Captain?" The answer is worthy of consideration by any aspirant to personality:

My belief concerning alcoholic beverages is beyond moderation or even temperance, I am a nonuser, and as such I do not feel that I am an unusual, queer individual who is out of step with the world. I find that there are many others who share this position with me. From my conversations with many people who do imbibe, I find that the majority of them wish that they did not.

Why do I refrain from drinking? The answer is simple: I cannot afford to drink.

Morally: I expect my children to grow up to be decent living adults. The only way to bring them up in the way they should go is to travel that way myself. When I realize that beverage alcohol is responsible for at least 37% pauperism and 45% of child destitution, and that more than 50% of the people in jail have been put there by alcohol, I conclude that "I can't afford to drink."

Financially: Maintaining a family of five, supporting my church and other charities, providing adequate insurance and continuing a sensible saving program, calls for discriminating judgment. To add an allowance for liquor would cause some other portion of the budget to suffer. Therefore "I can't afford to drink."

Socially: I know too many people who have worked hard to climb the difficult steps to success, and have lost it all during an evening of social drinking. I have not found an alcoholic yet who started out to be alcoholic. They all were going to be just "social drinkers," but in due time social drinking jeopardized their job, reputation, home and everything they had, and drinking became the ruling force of their life. "I can't afford to drink."

Physically: I still enjoy participating in active sports. I make the 25 mile road marches and 5 mile runs with my men without feeling the need of a "snort" to keep me going. I find that the majority of the outstanding champions will not touch liquor. I enjoy life. I want to live. "I can't afford to drink."

Very few military men have such a varied background as has Captain Keys. He won letters in high school football and track, he took special training in violin, voice, and trumpet, and he studied carpentry and agriculture. His chief current interest is serving with the paratroopers, 1st Airborne Battle Group, 501st Infantry, 101st Airborne Division, Fort Campell, Kentucky.

In our quest for personality, let's follow his example and resolve: "I cannot afford to drink/'

The following poem, "Someone Is Longing for a Perfect Gift," by Margaret Neel, is very much to the point:

He sends her red roses, with love in the note, Or a necklace of pearls for her tense lovely throat; He brings her rare treasures and tries hard to please; But the gift that she longs for is not one of these.

She would do without roses, their beauty and scent, For one special promise that was kept, and was meant; She would part with the pearls, so lustrous and fine, For one happy evening without taint and wine;

She would give up these presents of pleasure and pain For a small scrap of paper—his pledge to "Abstain."

A total abstainer, William Drees, the Netherlands Minister of the State, says:

A lasting basis for my conviction of abstinence is founded in the realization that alcohol, even when taken in small quantities, removes inner restraints and weakens self-control and self-mastery, so that consequently many persons who did not intend to go further than using alcohol to a moderate extent only end up by becoming victims of alcoholism.

And a writer in the *Christian Endeavor World* says:

Win your popularity by your pleasant personality, your skill in sports, your ability at dramatics or speaking. If you do these things and make friends easily, you will seldom have to worry about being unpopular just because you choose not to drink and smoke.

Alcohol is a retreat for weaklings from the miseries of their poor lives. It offers them no cures, only temporarily forgetfulness. It defeats their feeble efforts and makes their state worse than before. The craving for liquor and other stimulants, under the influence of which so much evil is done, is abnormal, a perverted compensation for lack of emotional life. A normal person in perfect health, full of zest and vitality, has no craving for alcohol. Certainly something is entirely wrong with a person's health and vitality if he feels the need of strong drink before he can get a "kick" out of life.

The Holy Scriptures call those who are deceived by strong drink unwise:

> Wine is a mocker, strong drink is raging:
> And whosoever is deceived thereby is not wise. (Prov. 20:1.)

> Who hath woe? who hath sorrow?
> Who hath contentions? who hath babbling?
> Who hath wounds without cause?
> Who hath redness of eyes?

>> They that tarry long at the wine;
>> They that go to seek mixed wine.

> Look not thou upon the wine when it is red,
> When it giveth his colour in the cup,
> When it moveth itself aright.

>> At the last it biteth like a serpent,
>> And stingeth like an adder. (Prov. 23:29-32.)

Do these words describe an individual who is a personality? Certainly not!

During World War I, I worked with the Army Post-mortem Corps. We labored under government orders in search of the then unknown bacilli that caused the Spanish influenza epidemic, which doctors were fighting. The Germans are known for their fondness for beer, and most all of those who came under our knives had been beer drinkers to some degree. According to the destruction of the inner organs, we classified them as occasional, customary, or heavy drinkers. We found kidneys more than ten times the normal size, and terribly deformed. Of course, the other organs were enlarged and deformed accordingly, and we wondered how it was possible that the once wonderful organs, now in this shape and condition, could do any work at all. Very often the exterior surface of the body—the drinker's nose, face, or neck—indicate the impairment and even the malfunction of the inner organs. The fact is that alcohol not only mars but destroys the physical and mental qualities of a personality. Alcohol and personality do not fit together. Therefore, avoid alcohol by all means, at all times, in any amount.

What should one do if one finds oneself in the grip of alcohol? Look for the nearest Alcoholics Anonymous group. They are fine people, with an understanding of your problems and weaknesses, because they have been successful in the same struggle. They will help you to overcome your problem. Go to them, and go right now!

If you have not started drinking, by all means don't start. That's the best guarantee against alcoholism and human misery. Seek the Lord, for He is always ready to give you the strength you need. This is the best surety for perfecting your personality. When tempted, always say proudly: "No thank you, I don't drink."

Let this be an expression of *your* personality.

12. LAWS OF NATURE AND PERSONALITY

"THEY SHALL walk with me in white: for they are worthy," said Jesus to the seer (Rev. 3:4). The worth of a personality is not reckoned in mathematical terms, but traced to the obedience or transgression of natural laws that God has established.

Through the agencies of nature, God is working day by day,

moment by moment, to keep us alive, to restore us to health, and to build us up to perfection.

Every habit that conflicts with the natural laws creates a diseased condition in body, soul, and spirit, and in proportion to the transgression physical suffering occurs. Body, soul, and spirit are enfeebled, and the personality marred.

Suffering follows transgression. Why? The first precept of nature's unfailing law reads: "Whatsoever a man soweth, that shall he also reap" (Gal. 6:7).

Here we have the explanation why 97 million people of the most prosperous nation in the world, the United States, are chronically ill, and also a revelation of the cause of all the ills and sufferings in the world. *All* those who transgress the laws of life and health, who abuse the stomach in gratifying lustful appetites, bear clear testimony to these transgressions in their bodies, and show the effects in their faces. Malformation of the body lines, sickness, disease of every kind, a ruined constitution, premature decay, and finally an untimely death are the results of the violation of natural laws. E. G. White says:

> If we unnecessarily injure our constitution, we dishonor God, for we transgress His laws of nature, the laws for our being and welfare. If appetite, which should strictly be guarded and controlled, is indulged as far as the injury of our body, the penalty of transgression will surely result.
>
> Those who understand something of the wisdom and beneficence of the laws of nature and perceive the evidence of God's love, and the blessings that result from obedience, will regard their duties and obligations (in regard to healthful living) from an altogether different point of view. Instead of looking upon the observance of the laws of health as a matter of sacrifice and self-denial, they will regard it as it is, an inestimable blessing.

Thomas M. Steger, in the *Journal of Natural Living*, tells us this:

> Sin punishes itself. When we disobey the traffic laws we may get away with it, because there is no officer there to arrest us at that time. However, the chronic offender will be caught sooner or

later, and as it is the case in some states, it means a loss of points, and continuous offenses will lead to suspension of the driver's license. When we disobey Nature's Laws either wilfully, or through our inherited ignorance or disregard of the truth, we suffer the same consequences. First, through acute, and, later on, chronic ailments. All during this time we have lost valuable points, and are on parole under suspended sentence, with the possibility of revocation of our tenure on life itself, because we have failed in one great purpose of life, and this is—to respect and to live up to God's Laws.

Dr. R. T. Trail, in his lecture "The True Healing Art" at the Smithsonian Institute, said:

Nature has not provided remedies for disease at all. She has provided penalties, not remedies. Disease is the consequence of a departure from physiological (natural) laws. There is no cure, except by a return to the obedience of the natural laws. The language of nature is the same as the language of the scripture: "The soul that sinneth shall die."

Look through nature up to nature's God, and realize the greatest truth of which the human mind is capable to conceive, that all, and through all, and with all, a loving Parent rules the universe, and that God is ultimately supreme. Health is found in obedience, and disease is the result of disobedience to His Laws.

Therefore, a careful conformity to the natural laws implanted in our being will insure health. We have no right to violate these principles of health and life, not even a single one. Ignorance and indifference in regard to these laws is dangerous, yet the violation of them is so common that people have come to look upon it with undue tolerance. That is a great mistake. Health and strength, vigor and vitality, charm and happiness, depend on close observance of the immutable laws. If you want health and not disease, youthfulness and not senility, longevity and not premature death, inform yourself in regard to these laws of life and health, return to the obedience of them, and live in conformity with them.

Charm, beauty, vitality, and a youthful personality are gifts of nature for those who live according to its laws. This is the best formula for living a happy and pleasant life up to a youthful golden age.

13.   HABITS AND PERSONALITY

We sow our thoughts, and we reap our actions;
We sow our actions, and we reap our habits;
We sow our habits, and we reap our character;
We sow our character, and we reap our destiny.

Nothing is stronger than habit. More than anything else, food habits can make or break a personality, physically and mentally.

Many people, instead of "eating to live," simply 'live to eat." There is a very great difference. Those who live to eat ignore two great laws, the laws of moderation and temperance. Sooner or later, nature exacts penalties for violating one or the other of these, her cardinal laws. Most of our physical ills, and a considerable proportion of our spiritual trials, are the consequence of transgressions of these laws of nature. Great cities, even entire nations, like Nineveh, Babylon, Greece, and Rome, have ended in oblivion because of these violations and transgressions.

What and how to eat are immensely important matters, far more important than is generally recognized. Not only do they involve the building of personality, but the health, happiness, existence, and the very destiny of humanity as well.

Eating should be more than a matter of pleasant satisfaction, it should also be a thoughtful, considered function. Everything we do in life should be done for a definite purpose. And so should eating. After all, eating is the most important thing we do in life, from the cradle to the grave, is it not?

Whatever calling we fulfill in life, whatever we do, primarily we do it to sustain life, of which the major portion is eating.

Does this sound too materialistic? Nevertheless, it is the truth.

In our business and in our social life we observe many general laws, and we are very careful to follow good rules. But do we observe good rules in the most important, the most interesting function of our life—eating? Are we concerned? Do we observe laws and rules? Oh, no. Many of us know very little about the most simple, most necessary laws of eating. We do not ask ourselves why we eat, what we should eat, and what we should not eat, and we do not care what the consequences may be.

The *National Health Review* reports that more than seventy million Americans suffer from deficiencies of one kind or another. This does not necessarily mean that they lack a sufficient supply of food. On the contrary, many of these sufferers have plenty of what they call "good food." It does not indicate this at all. But it does indicate, and demonstrate very clearly, that their intake of food is unbalanced and, chemically, inharmoniously combined. It further demonstrates ignorance or carelessness in the most important matter of our physical life—the matter of eating.

In building and maintaining our physical personality, three fundamental laws must be considered and cannot be ignored.

1. *Select* only the right food for eating, the kinds that contain the necessary sixteen elements of which the body consists. (See chapter 7 which gives the sources of nutrients.)

2. *Combine* only the right kinds of food for eating, the kinds that chemically harmonize when combined.

3. *Balance* the diet, and proportion your meals according to the elements as nearly as possible. Do not overserve some elements and underserve others. It is true that some housewives can do more for the health and welfare of their families than half a dozen doctors, and it is equally true that other housewives do more for doctors than their families.

Transgressions of these fundamental laws will result in abnormal conditions, in weakness, disease, and premature old age. Meditate right here on a nation that is rich in everything, yet contains more than seventy million people with physical deficiencies. What is the cause? You should find the answer easily.

Obedience to and strict enforcement of these rules will result in health, vigor, happiness, and youthful longevity. The more closely these laws are obeyed, the more harmonious will be the development and maintenance of your body. There will be more resistance against the enemies of life, and a better and higher unfolding of your physical personality.

As long as people eat and drink incorrectly, pay no attention to right food habits, are heedless of the poisoning and devitalizing of their food supplies, live under artificial conditions, and dine on artificially treated foods, they will have to contend with weakness, disease, unhappiness, and premature old age.

Man has been trained through the ages to believe that disease is a tangible thing that can be cured by drugs, and that youth and longevity can be gotten by some magical potion. This is an unreasonable superstition. In the light of modern medicine, there is no cure, only relief, whereas, in the light of true science, curing an ailment is possible in only one way, and that is by removing the cause.

The cause in most of these millions of deficiency cases is disobedience to nature's laws, the violation of the laws of nutrition. Therefore, strict obedience to these laws is the only way to restore, build up, and maintain that wonderful human body. There is no other way. Consider again that report on the nation's health: 71,000,000 people suffering because of deficiencies; 91,000,000 sick within one year; 45 per cent of our young men rejected after medical examination as unfit for the armed services, and so on. What does this report tell us?

Habit has made the world's greatest nation a land full of faulty physical personalities. Habitual violation of the laws of nature shows up in the soured ones, the half alive, and the living dead.

Practically, believe it or not, it is very easy for nearly all these people to be changed into real, happy, charming personalities, if they only would be willing to alter their habits. Habits are stronger than nature, therefore change your habits and start *today*. Ovid wrote:

> Habits gather by unseen degrees,
> As brooks make rivers,
> And rivers run to the sea.

Wrong habits may develop to such a degree that gradually and surely they will destroy health, happiness, and personality. They are a constituent that can add or subtract from your personality. Will you decide to cope with your habits?

May I remind you that in personality engineering each of us is his own "supreme court/' each of us must use his own intelligence, his own reasoning, and his own will power in making the final decision in this matter.

Now, analyze your eating and living habits. Make two columns. One for right habits, the other for wrong habits. There is absolutely no third column. What you cannot set down under the heading "Right Habits" must go under "Wrong Habits," whether you like it or not. Be honest with yourself. It will bring you great dividends. You may not finish this analysis right away, but you can start it now. And as you check a habit, evaluate it in the light and knowledge you have gained, and place it in the proper column.

Lessons must be learned in self-control, self-denial, and temperance. True temperance teaches us to dispense entirely with everything hurtful to our well-being. Very few people realize how much their eating habits have to do with their usefulness, loveliness, character, personality, and eternal destiny.

Moral and intellectual power must rule, not appetite. The body must be the servant of the mind, not vice versa. Every habit that injures the body's health reacts unfavorably upon the mind. Anything that lessens physical strength enfeebles the mind, makes it less capable of discriminating between right and wrong, less capable of choosing the good, and gives it less strength to do what is right.

Do not say: "Oh, please don't tell me that I shouldn't smoke, miss my cocktail, or abstain from this or that. I know it's bad, but I just love it, and I don't want to change."

This is a pitiful protest often uttered by victims of wrong habits. Such people show a lack of will power to analyze their troubles impartially, a lack of courage to deal with their weaknesses properly.

Thus we are happy or miserable in accordance with our daily habits, and thus we make or unmake our personality.

According to John Dryden, "We first make our habits, then our habits make us." And N. Emmons says: "Habits are either the worst of masters, or the best of servants." Never be slow to break bad habits of eating or others. Unless bad habits are conquered, they will conquer us, and destroy our present and eternal happiness.

Wrong habits cannot be taken to heaven. The precious hours of probation (our life) are granted us so that we may overcome and remove bad habits, and then form others that will build a personality that is useful in this life and fit for heaven.

Take your stand. Cultivate right habits under all circumstances. If you feel that terrific power of temptation and that drawing desire that leads to indulgence, do not say: "I cannot resist." You can if you will. Have faith in God. He has already provided help for you to overcome.

When Adam and Eve yielded to their intemperate appetites, they lost their blissful Eden, and life eternal. But Christ, in His great love to save man, came and withstood the fiercest temptation, overcame appetite, and restored Eden, to give life eternal back to all who are willing to overcome. "To him that over-cometh will I grant to sit with me in my throne, even as I also overcame, and am set down with my Father in his throne" (Rev. 3:21).

If you will not call Christ a liar, believe this promise, and He will give you strength to overcome *all* bad habits, and this promise will be yours.

The following quotations are taken from the writings of that notable reformer, E. G. White. They merit careful study by all who are engaged in personality engineering. Christian virtues consist of good and right habits. It is habit that makes or breaks your personality.

If the appetite is allowed to rule, the mind will be brought under its control. Those who are slaves to appetite will fail in perfecting a Christian character. Christ began his work of redemption by reforming the physical habits of man.

The tobacco habit frequently affects the nervous system in a more powerful manner than does the use of alcohol. Body and mind are in many cases more thoroughly intoxicated with the use of tobacco, than with spirituous liquors; for it is a more suitable poison.

The liquor habit enfeebles the intellect, and the moral powers are weakened. The sensibilities are benumbed, the claims of God and heaven are not realized, eternal things are not appreciated. The Bible declares that no drunkard shall inherit the kingdom of God.

Through the habit of overeating the foundation of the human machinery is gradually undermined, the power of the brain is lessened, the brain nerve energy is benumbed and almost paralyzed. Intemperance in eating, even of food of the right quality, will have a prostrating influence upon the system. . . . Strict temperance in eating and drinking is highly essential for the healthy preservation and vigorous use of all the functions of the body. The stomach must have careful attention. It must not be kept in continual operation. Give this misused and much-abused organ some rest. With proper food and regular habits the stomach will gradually recover.

The pernicious habit of self-abuse is, in many cases, the only real cause of the numerous complaints of the young. Headache, catarrh, dizziness, nervousness, pain in the shoulders and side, loss of appetite, pain in the back and the limbs, wakeful, feverish nights, tired feelings in the morning and great exhaustion after exercising, beauty of health disappearing, and marked sallow countenance. Have you been aroused sufficiently to look beneath the surface, to inquire into the cause of this physical decay?

Industrious habits must be a part of the education given to the youth. We need schools to educate children and youth that they may be masters of labor, and not slaves of labor. The habit of industry will be found an important aid to the youth in resisting temptation.

We are not excusable if through ignorance we destroy God's building by taking into the stomach poisonous drugs under varied names we do not understand.

Drug medication, as it is practiced generally, is a curse. Educate away from drugs, use them less and less, and depend more upon hygienic agencies.

Nature will respond to God's remedies—pure air, pure water, proper exercise, and a clear conscience.

To use drugs while continuing evil habits is certainly inconsistent, and greatly dishonors God by dishonoring the body He made. The use of tea, coffee, tobacco, opium, wine, beer, and other stimulants gives nature false support.

The physician who endeavors to enlighten his patients as to the nature and cause of their troubles and maladies, and to teach them how to avoid disease, may have uphill work; but if he is a conscientious reformer, he will talk plainly to his patients of the ruinous effects of self-indulgence in eating and drinking, of the overtaxation of the vital forces that has brought his patients where they are. He will not increase the evil by administering drugs till exhausted nature gives up the struggle, but will teach his patients how to form correct habits to aid nature in her work of restoration, by wise use of her own simple remedies.

14. BEAUTY AND PERSONALITY

> Beautiful in form and feature,
> Lovely as the day,
> Can there be so fair a creature,
> Formed of common clay?
>
> CHORUS OF THE GRACES

> The light of love—the purity of grace,
> The mind—the music breathing from her face,
> The heart, whose softness harmonized the whole,
> And oh! the eye was in itself a soul.
>
> BRIDE OF ABYDOS

Beauty, Beautiful. These terms mean to excel in form and feature, to arouse esthetic pleasure, to be charming and delightful. They imply wholesomeness of body and soul, softness of outline, and delicacy of mold. They are opposed to everything artificial, hard, and rugged.

Handsome, Fair. These terms are inferior to beautiful, but denote what is bright, smooth, clear, and without blemish.

Picturesque. This term is often used for made-up qualities expressing ornamentation, having pictorial value.

Make-up. This term is used for costumes, wigs, and cosmetics, and to assume a theatrical role. It also is used for lipstick, powder, rouge, etc., applied to a woman's face and nails, on hands and feet.

THE ABOVE definitions are taken from the New Standard Dictionary, to render it easier to evaluate and estimate the real worth of beauty and to understand clearly the meaning of the noun "beauty" and the adjective "beautiful."

After you have studied these definitions carefully, I believe you will join the writer wholeheartedly in agreeing with Homer, the epic poet of Greece, who said: "Beauty is a glorious gift of nature."

Further, I believe you will agree that the adjective and modifier "skin-deep" you find in the dictionary cannot be an attribute of "beauty," but it is appropriately used with make-up. In other words, beauty implies wholesomeness; make-up is applied skin-deep.

Every trait of beauty may be referred to some virtue, such as innocence, candor, generosity, modesty, and so on. If men and women would only realize the full power of real personal beauty!

I hear you say: "I am not beautiful, so I must help myself. I want to have rosy cheeks, inviting red lips . . . Are they not called the gateway to the soul, and the outlet of the heart? I don't have them, therefore I ..."

Very well, but learn the right way, the natural, the deep, the real way. Then you will be blessed with real beauty from inside out, with beauty that lasts. Then you may forget the artificial, skin-deep way, a way by which you drive away real beauty. Beauty begs you to take her. She is conditionally available for everyone. What are the conditions? They are two: {a) adherence to nature's immutable laws of life, headed by the law of nutrition, and (b) the cherishing of noble thoughts, hopes, and purposes. It is the divinity within that makes the divinity without, that is, beauty.

In the second volume of this work, "Your Personality—the Soul," we shall study and elaborate further on the beauty of the soul. In this chapter we shall dwell only on nature's methods of beautifying "Your Personality—the Body."

We shall discuss some beauty secrets that bring real and sure results, which will truly improve our physical personality. I say "beauty secrets," not make-up secrets. The difference is vast, and the results incomparably different. The word "make-up" implies something artificial, something that should be there but is missing. Now, let us focus our eyes on what is missing. What is it? Real beauty!

COLORFUL   PERSONALITY

A colorful personality is one that is full of contrasting color, full of temperament, vivid, exciting, inspiring. Your personality also requires such colorfulness for its physical part—the body. Professor Julius Gilbert White, author of Abundant Health, declares :

> There is an unalterable relation between the physical, mental, and spiritual phases of human experience. For any one of these three to be normal, all three must advance in co-ordinate unision. Only in this way can man reach his own highest ideal, and the eminence intended by his Maker.

The words "beautiful" and "colorful" are synonymous, similar in meaning, and alike in significance. They describe conditions that abound in contrast, such as starry, sparkling eyes, complexion, color hue or the appearance of the skin, especially of the face, gleaming pink cheeks, and enticing red lips. Add this to a streamlined body with correct poise and posture and you have the fundamentals for a physical personality par excellence.

This is not a course in mannerisms, or in sitting, walking, or talking techniques, but simply the fundamental rules to follow and habits to establish in the pursuit of a colorful, radiant personality.

THE   SKIN

In regard to beauty, first attention must be given to the skin, its texture and disposition. One should look for, and eradicate, any blemish that may mar and destroy its beauty and colorful-ness.

Shakespeare declared: "A beautiful skin must be as smooth and as transparent as monumental alabaster." And that is what our Maker planned the human skin to be. That is also what nature needs to beautify our body, "a clear, blemishless transparent skin." It is the canvas on which the great artist, nature, paints in the highlights on a colorful physical personality.

The skin is a marvelous covering. It weighs one eighth of a person's body weight, or about twenty pounds for a person who weighs 160 pounds, and it has an average surface of about sixteen square feet. Thousands of miles of arteries and very small blood vessels called capillaries run through it, producing that pretty, rosy hue. And there are thousands of miles of sensory nerves along the surface—the telegraph wires and stations— ceaselessly conveying messages to the H.Q., always tattling to central everything that is going on around the outside of their inside world.

Presuming we are in a hot desert and able to listen to their conversation, we would probably hear something like this: "We cannot stand this terrible heat, H.Q. Cannot anything be done about it?" Right away, the H.Q. gives two orders. One is to the sweat glands, asking them to get rid of all the water they can. Promptly, sweat begins to exude lavishly and profusely, and from two to five quarts a day is discharged. The other order goes to the capillaries in the surface of the skin, asking them to enlarge their caliber to permit more hot blood to come to the surface. This too is promptly obeyed. The small blood vessels enlarge, more blood comes to the surface, more heat is thrown off, and the skin becomes a deeper, prettier hue of red. If we were in the High Sierras or Alaska, where there is much snow and ice, we could also hear the conversation, but with opposite orders and results.

The skin is a protective leather jacket. Because of this, it is permeated and impregnated with a very valuable substance, a highly insoluble, albuminous chemical compound called keratin, which resists almost all natural solvents, such as water, oil, acids, alkalis, and other liquid chemicals. Nothing from outside can permeate the skin to harm the inside cell life, not even one drop of water. If the skin were not like this, imagine what might happen when you took a bath and water permeated the skin to the inner body. Shall we not gratefully join King David in saying, "I will praise thee; for I am fearfully and wonderfully made: marvellous are thy works; and that my soul knoweth right well" (Ps. 139:14).

There are more than 3,000,000 pores in your skin, or about 2,000 to every square inch, and in the palms of the hands and the soles of the feet there are more than double that amount. For what purpose?

SEWAGE OUTLETS

The pores are necessary because the skin, with its sweat-gland system, is one of the four sewage outlets of the body. The others are the bowels, the kidneys, with the urinary system, and the lungs, with the respiratory system.

The pores are the openings of the sweat glands. These are little spiral tubes from one-fourth to one-third of an inch in length. It is estimated that if they could be put together, end to end, it would show that this sewage system is about fifteen miles long, with a surface covering of about 5,000 square feet.

Imagine three million sewage outlets for toxins from inside your body. Scientists tell us that the daily output is never less than two pints of poison-laden vapor, all of which passes through these microscopic sewers. In dry heat it may be as much as ten pints per day. Normally, we may not be consciously aware of this, except in hot weather, when we perspire a great deal, because perspiration generally evaporates as fast as the body throws it off. But there is refuse left after evaporation that very readily becomes rancid. It is this rancidity that gives the peculiar tainted smell to underwear and parts of the body. Frequent changes of underwear and regular bathing are essentials in our personality engineering. The nostrils detect the non-bather just as readily as the smoker and the drinker.

The most marvelous thing is that in a lifetime the body eliminates not less than 32,000 quarts of water and sewage through the skin, yet not even a drop of water can permeate the skin from the outside. The Heavenly Engineer designed and built into the skin a perfect mechanism for one-way traffic only, and a leakage has never been found.

The skin is a sunshade, a protection against the actinic rays from outer space. It protects the delicate cells from harm by deadly ultraviolet and other rays. For this reason, the skin manufactures a chemical called melanin, which causes the forming of a summer tan that blocks out harmful rays.

The skin also is provided with a marvelous insulator and thermostatic system to regulate the temperature and to keep out extreme heat and cold. Our skin is amazingly and wonderfully made. What are you doing to keep it healthy and beautiful?

Remember, the elasticity of your skin will show your real age, that is, the physiological, in contrast to the chronological age. Are you feeling old when you should still be young?

Know this: all eruptions, blemishes, and so-called skin diseases, from blackheads and pimples to smallpox and cancer, are caused by impure blood, by inner uncleanliness, and by faulty elimination of body-waste toxins. It is nature's method of eliminating morbid matter, of throwing out toxins from within.

Decay of any kind within the body gives rise to toxins of a damaging nature, and it is the function of the bowels, the kidneys, the lungs, and the skin to eliminate these poisons from the system. The *Good Health Journal* reports that cancer specialists throughout the world have come to the conclusion that there is some very close connection between cancer and general systemic poisoning resulting from bowel toxins generated by putrefactive bacteria.

Dr. Lane, an eminent London surgeon, believes that constipation and toxemia, resulting from putrefaction in the colon, is the chief cause of cancer.

Dr. A. C. Jordan, in his presidential address before the British Medical Society, declared:

> In chronic intestinal stasis, active pathogenic bacteria thrive in the bowels. These form poisonous products in the intestines, which are carried by way of the thoracic duct into the general circulation, and thus reach every living cell in the body. No

tissue or organ can resist their baleful influence; every tissue attached by them loses some of its power of resistance to pathogenic influences; and this lowered resistance has a very potent influence in favoring the occurrence of cancer.

Microbiologist J. Empringham declares:

The lower bowel of the average person is continually dominated by billions of putrefactive bacteria that are constantly generating poisons. It is estimated that the average person expels over thirty trillions of bacteria germs from the colon every day. More than one third by weight of the feces is made up of these microbes, too small to be seen unless magnified at least four hundred diameters.

Many kinds of bacteria gain entrance to the lower bowel in food residue, and more than a hundred species are known to flourish there, whenever permitted to do so.

ELIMINATION

In the quest for health and beauty, the most perplexing problem and one of the least understood, is that of eliminating the body wastes. It is a case of ignorance, "out of sight, out of mind," and this ignorance is the number-one killer in our country.

The fact is that all body wastes are toxic. These toxins are harmless as long as they are promptly eliminated from the body by the natural channels. But if they are restrained (by constipation, for instance) they become extremely harmful, causing loss of vigor and vitality, beauty and charm, health and finally life.

How greatly important the heavenly Architect considered this matter of elimination can readily be seen from the fact that he provided *four* avenues of elimination—bowels, kidneys, lungs, and the skin—but only *one* for reception—the mouth. (If there is any question about the lungs being an organ of reception— which they are, be assured, for air—let us state that the subject will be dealt with fully in Volume III of this series. Here we discuss only the receiving of food into the body and the elimination of its residue.)

In our personality engineering we have found that very great care is necessary in selecting the things that shall enter into our body through the mouth. Now we shall learn that still greater consideration must be given to the matter of the wastes that shall leave our body by elimination.

There are two distinctive types of body waste to consider: digestive waste, and catabolic waste. If these wastes are not readily eliminated, they create a condition in the body known as systemic poisoning, or toxemia, which is considered the general cause of all blemishes, all kinds of diseases, and premature old age.

Now, let us take a close look at digestive waste, which is the cause of constipation and a great trouble maker in many a life. In a former chapter we followed the food from the table to the small intestine. There the prepared nutritive portion of the food was sucked up by the millions of villi suction pumps, and loaded onto the moving cafeteria, the blood stream, for general distribution. The largest portion of the food was left in the small intestine as refuse, or residue. Let us see what happens to that.

Continued peristaltic movements—let us call them mass movements—push the mass of residue toward the intersection of the small and the large intestine, or the colon. The H.Q. orders the gatekeeper to open the gate. His name is ileocecal valve, or ileocoli. With prompt obedience the gate is opened, permitting the passage of the refuse into the lower pouch of the colon, called the caecum. And here is where mankind's greatest trouble starts.

Civilization's most widespread malady is constipation, which is inward uncleanliness, inward filthiness. This is not a disease, it is *the* disease.

The different ailments are only nature's varied efforts to throw the accumulated toxins out of the body, to eliminate. This is true, from a simple pimple to smallpox and cancer.

Much has been written pro and con about constipation by physicians and laity alike. Still the matter is very little understood, in fact, people are much confused about it.

Constipatus is a Latin word that means to press together, stopping or preventing passage. *Constipation*, the English equivalent, is understood to mean that the colon is filled with hard-pressed feces, and evacuations are few and difficult. It is all this indeed, plus autointoxication and toxemia with all its manifold complications. Billions of dollars are spent yearly by the American people to relieve this condition in various ways. But it appears that the more civilized we become, the more laxatives we need.

The lower bowel, or colon, is shaped like a capital U turned upside down. The refuse of digestion from the small intestine enters this sewer near the bottom, at the right-hand side of the body, and in consequence the fecal matter must climb uphill for nearly one foot, in the ascending colon. For this reason the cecum, the blind pouch below the ileocecal valve, which is the lowest part of the ascending colon, is the chief seat of constipation. It is here that the fecal matter collects, just as rubbish sinks and accumulates at the bottom of a well or pool.

Wilfred Hill, in *The Living Stream*, says: "The first thing I learned by experience and which, ever since I understood it, has been a basic factor in keeping me fit... was the vital importance of inward cleanliness and the natural elimination of waste toxins from the body."

J. Empringham urges that we conquer constipation nature's way—all purgatives are poisons. Castor oil, epsom salts, jalap, magnesia, senna, cascara, phenolphthalein, rhubarb, podophyllin, aloes, and all the *harmless* (?) vegetable and herbal laxatives are habit-forming and injurious, he points out. To move regularly, frequently, and naturally, the bowel flora must be dominated by native B acidophilus. Moreover, in order that putrefactive bacteria traveling through the gastrointestinal tract in food residue may not have time to penetrate and multiply in the lower intestine, the bowel must be supplied with enough *bulk, moisture,* and *lubrication* to cause several natural evacuations each day, he adds.

"A lack of any one of these three things invariably brings about constipation. Unfortunately, most of the food that passes through the digestive machinery of civilized people is deficient in all of these qualities, and the inevitable result is that the refuse becomes impacted and decomposed in the lower bowel, and converts the colon into a seething cesspool of poison," he concludes.

Volumes could be written on the subject, but a few quotations and recommendations may suffice for our purpose. The cause is misunderstanding and ignorance of this very important matter of life and living. Dr. Walker expressed the situation aptly in a poem entitled "Constipation" in his book *Are You Slipping*?

> The days of your health would surely be
>   Shorter by far and fewer,
> If you lived in a house where there could be
>   A stopped up or clogged up sewer.
>
> But the state of your health must ever be faced,
>   If you carry wherever you go,
> At work or play, the corruption and waste
>   That's been with you from long, long ago.
>
> We can't look inside, so we are not aware
>   That the colon needs constant attention,
> When neglected, we're sick, and then we don't dare
>   To ascribe it to colon retention.
>
> When a person has natural movements each day,
>   It's a source of much irritation
> To be told that his ailments are carried away
>   By a colonic good irrigation.
>
> It's a recognized fact, beyond doubt or debate,
>   That the colon, cesspool of the body,
> When cleaned out in time and not left till too late
>   Saves more lives than prescriptions more gaudy.

> So, my friend, face the fact while you're still here to stay,
>   Don't depend on your imagination.
> Do what thousands of others are doing today—
>   Go and get a colon irrigation.

He continues:

One of the dangers of letting waste matter accumulate in the colon is absorption, principally while we sleep, of poisons which are generated as a result of putrefaction.

Carbolic acid is one and indol is another. These two are probably the most serious, as they result in headache and lassitude to begin with, and may develop into biliousness (liver trouble), paralysis of the intestines, and peritonitis (inflammation of the serous membrane that lines the abdominal cavity). A deficiency of hydrochloric acid secretion (the stomach digestive fluid) also is a condition resulting from this presence of indol.

Microbiologist J. Empringham, renowned authority on intestinal research, declares:

Intestinal toxemia is frequently due to the unfortunate fact that the putrefying mass of corruption in the lower bowel often returns into the small intestine.

This cannot happen normally, because the small intestine is separated from the colon by a trapdoor, or valve, which is designed to open only one way. This is called the ileocecal valve.

When the wastes of digestion are permitted to remain longer than necessary, or naturally, in the colon, excessive putrefaction takes place. The irritating poisons generated by toxic bacteria inflame and degenerate the membrane, especially the delicate mechanism of the ileocecal valve, with the result that the trapdoor gets out of commission, permitting the poisonous sewage of the colon to leak back into the small intestine.

Now the walls of the small intestine enable liquid to pass through them into the blood stream. The result is that, when poisonous matter from the colon sewer backs up into the small intestine, the toxin rapidly passes into the blood, causing general systemic poisoning, ill health, and old age.

Suggestions that have been followed (or the moral accepted) with gratifying results include Dr. W. N. Walker's recipe to become constipated, published in Become Younger:

> The greatest friend of a constipated colon is starchy food. Starches are the most prolific media for the propagation of gas forming bacteria. If I wanted to generate volumes of gas in my system I would start with toast (white, whole wheat, soy, or any kind) or hot cake for breakfast, donuts and coffee for lunch, and noodles, spaghetti, cake, etc., for dinner. I know I also would become beautifully constipated on such food. Furthermore, I know perfectly well that on such food I would never expect to become younger.

Another formula to lose beauty and health, and to become constipated: drink plenty of tea and coffee, if possible with your meals, and you can be sure of earning a sorrowful harvest.

Tea and coffee cannot be classified as foods. They are drugs, very harmful and habit forming. Tea, coffee, cocoa, and chocolate all contain the same or closely allied elements. The exhilarating effects are equally as great as are the anesthetic effects of other drugs. For instance, in South America the use of the cocoa leaf is very common. The chronic cocoa eater can always be recognized by his appearance—hollow eyes, sunken cheeks, trembling hands, mental depression, and so on. And so it is with the chronic coffee or tea drinker.

Dr. Adolphus Hohensee, a noted health lecturer and authority on healthful living, enumerates the results of the use of tea and coffee as follows:

Indigestion	Palpitation of the heart
Headache	Muscular lassitude
Insomnia	Degeneration of the kidneys,
Sallow skin	liver, and arteries
Irritated nerves	Constipation
Irritated temper	Temporary high blood pressure
Shaking hands	Permanent high blood pressure
Poisoned blood stream	Anemia
	Apoplexy

He goes on to say:

> These are the conditions science has shown to come to us from the use of tea and coffee. No doubt, many of you are fond of these drinks, are wedded to them, and perhaps slaves to them. You may have to fight to get free, but you should do it, and you should start today and stick to it until you win, because you are in a terrible bondage which will be your undoing.
>
> You have no idea how much better you will feel a month from now if you will utterly abandon these practices. You may say this is hard to believe, because your grandmother drank tea and coffee all her life. I cannot help it if she did; these are the facts nevertheless, and you would do well to listen.

Jethro Kloss, sharing his lifetime experiences in his work *Back to Eden*, states: "Nearly the entire race is afflicted with constipation. Waste matter is left entirely too long in the body." Among the causes of constipation, he gives wrong diet as the main one, and eating foods that do not contain enough roughage or bulk, and foods that are devitalized. He also names the following: lack of muscular tone in the bowels, improper mastication of food, a meat diet, too many varieties of food at one meal, coffee, tea, and liquor of all kinds, irregular habits of attending to the call of nature, a sedentary life, and lack of exercise.

"These are contributing factors to this universal ailment. The life-giving properties which would aid digestion are removed from the food we eat, or are spoiled by improper cooking and wrong combination. Excessive use of drugs and patent medicines is another frequent cause of constipation" he concludes.

Constipating foods are white flour, white rice, blackberries, boiled milk, barley, brown flour gruel, brown flour gravy, fried foods, all processed cheese, all kinds of meat, boiled eggs, and starchy products.

Constipation can be prevented (or relieved) by observing the following suggestions:

Regulate the diet.

Eat your food as dry as possible. (If the food is eaten dry and thoroughly saturated with saliva, it is a wonderful help in lubrieating the bowels. It makes the system alkaline, and greatly increases the rapidity of digestion.)

Do your drinking one hour before or after meals. Drinking with meals is very harmful.

Eat freely of fresh fruits, such as apples, figs, peaches, oranges, bananas, and blueberries.

Fruits and vegetables should not be eaten at the same meal.

Visit the toilet regularly after each meal to train the bowels.

Food should digest readily. Waste matters should be eliminated promptly.

This Fruit Delight laxative is recommended by Dr. H. J. Walch:

1 lb. prunes (seeded)	1 lb. figs
1 lb. raisins	1 cup raw bran

Run the fruit through the food chopper and then mix it with the bran. Form into squares containing a tablespoonful to the square and wrap in waxed paper like candy kisses. Eat one Fruit Delight each day.

This is a most excellent laxative. The raw bran contains a special enzyme found in raw milk and raw bran, and so far as is known is not found elsewhere. This helps to normalize the digestive tract and makes elimination natural and normal.

Dr. Walker advises the taking of a series of cleansing colonies, plus the following:

The colon of any person who has lived all his life eating processed, cooked, and canned foods cannot possibly be free from an accumulation of waste and corruption in the colon. To enable the colon to function properly, its nerves and muscles must necessarily be up to par. Proper nourishment, consisting mainly of plenty of fresh raw vegetables and fruits and their juices, can take care of this situation naturally. Carrot and spinach juice, fresh and raw, is the finest organic nourishment for it.

The story of vanishing beauty and encroaching infirmity, senility, and old age is the story of autointoxication and toxemia.

The toxin of body waste is the only culprit guilty of all outer blemishes.

The toxin of body waste is the only cause of vanishing beauty.

The toxin of body waste is the final cause of all diseases and infection.

The toxin of body waste is the only cause of senility and old age.

The toxin of body waste is the main cause of premature death.

An arterial system composed of many thousands of miles of elastic hose from one twenty-five thousandths of an inch to one inch in diameter reaches every tissue, every particle of skin, yes, every single cell in our wonderful body. Thousands of miles of this hose are laid throughout the skin.

Blood, the great mystery of life that no scientist has yet been able to solve, is the great depository of all our body's constructive forces. It also is the collector and transportation agent of all toxins and destructive elements, the waste products of the body.

All procedures for health and beauty in personality engineering must begin here, and nowhere else. If you are determined to build your personality, you must co-operate with your Maker, the "great I AM," keep your body free from every kind of toxin and poison, and eat only the right kind and the right amount of food.

Do this and you may be assured that the great heavenly appointed artist within you, whose name is blood, will rebuild every organ, gland, tissue, and all cells back to normal. He will mold for you a lovely form, create sparkling eyes and a smooth alabaster-like skin, paint lovely pink cheeks and enticing red lips—yes, if you will co-operate he will naturally beautify *your personality, the body.*

15. YOUTHFULNESS AND PERSONALITY

YOUTHFULNESS is the goal of personality engineering. There is a truth in the old saying that "those whom the gods love die young," meaning that they keep their youthfulness until the very end, even to a ripe old age. It seems to me that it would be more truthful and meaningful if the saying were changed to read: "Those who love God die young."

Why is it that in our present age so many people grow old when they are still young? What is amiss?

A little boy once spoke a great truth when his teacher asked him: "Sonny, what will you be when you are grown up?"
"Alive, alive, professor," came the quick reply.

Oh, what a wonderful answer! Alive! alive! To be alive is one of the most important personality traits. A jovial philosopher expounded: "Too many people exist only; they die when they are but 25 or 30 years old, and then wait until they are 70 or 80 to be buried." A great truth, and philosophy indeed.

Who wants to be a real personality cannot only exist; he must be alive, full of pep, of vim and vigor, of health and youthfulness. This does not mean merely to be free from pain and discomfort; it means to be in possession of and to exercise vigor and vitality.

The desire of the ages has been longevity, and through history we can follow a long, long throng of hunters for the elixir of life. Of course, their dreams have not been of longevity only, but of long-lasting youthfulness. It would be a calamity if longevity only lengthened the period of old age, weakness, senility, and misery. If the infirmities of old age remain, longevity is not worth seeking. Let the weary and worn go to their well-earned rest. Only the physical, mental, and spiritual qualities of youthfulness—these attributes of personality—give us a right to live longer.

Oliver Wendell Holmes said: "To be seventy years young is sometimes far more cheerful and hopeful than to be forty years old."

And Lord Lloyd, speaking about the explorer, Aurel Stein, declared: "The farther he goes, the younger he grows."

We like the story of the elderly lady with the lovely complexion and the small boy who asked her: "Please, madam, are you old or young?"

"My dear," said the lady, "I have been young a very long time."

Let us be young a long, long time. Of course, you cannot postpone birthdays. Senescence is nature's way, but you must not accept senility as a matter of course. Senescence comes from the Latin senesco, meaning senior, to be aged in years, while senility means physical and mental infirmity. This is not in the plan of our Creator; it is a technique of the old arch-killer, who was a murderer from the beginning. Let us rather follow the 82-year-old preacher, H. E. Fosdick, joyously shouting: "It's magnificent to grow old if one keeps young."

Personality means youthfulness, and do you know that you can grow to be one hundred and twenty years of age and still be youthful, with all the charm, vigor, vitality, and qualities of youth?

Years ago, in Europe, I found a list of more than 300 Bulgarian centenarians. One hundred and fourteen of them had passed the 120-year mark. In the Tibetan borderland of the Hunzas, centenarians in full manhood are very common. Barbara Pataleewa, the renowned Soviet writer, relates that on the slopes of the Himalayas, she shared a simple meal with two young Indians. When she asked their age (in the Far East it is very polite to ask, "What is your honorable age?") she was amazed to learn that one was 116 and the other 119 years young.

Once, when traveling in the mountains of eastern Tibet, I joined two pilgrims who were on their way to one of the holy shrines to Buddha. The older one, already several weeks on the road and still strong of foot, had with him his "baby," as he called his son. When I asked, according to Chinese polite custom, their "honorable age," I learned that the "baby" was 78 and the elder was 102 years young.

One time, I had the privilege of exchanging the "rite of humility" with an apparently young man in the little church of Waterford, in central California. He not only was physically but also mentally full of vim and vigor. The pastor of that church was about to be transferred to another one, and at the farewell meeting this "young" man went with steady steps to the rostrum, and gave a wonderfully clear recital of a poem he had composed for the occasion. And his age? He had recently celebrated his 106th birthday.

The stories of the young Count de Saint Germain are many. Here is just one. At a luncheon in the palace at Versailles, the handsome count, who seemed to be in his late thirties, was conversing with the aged Comtesse De George. Her husband had been French ambassador to Italy about a half century before. "But surely, Monsieur," said the old lady, "I met your father in Venice, in the year 1710." (This was about 1760.) "No, Comtesse, it was I whom you met on that occasion." To convince her, he related many little incidents of the meeting, of how he danced, flirted, and played games with her. Yes, with the appearance of a man in the thirties, the handsome count was a centenarian.

The beautiful Ninon de Lenclos was charmingly coquettish at the age of 82. The story goes that two cavaliers, neither of them more than thirty, resorted to pistols in a duel to decide whose sweetheart the 82-year-young beauty should be.

Some years ago, a European newspaper reported: "A 93-year-young Polish mother has given birth to a 7-pound baby girl. Mother and daughter are fine."

Dr. Alfred C. Kinsey, in *Sexual Behavior in the American Male,* noted that a Chicago husband, 89, and his wife, 91, enjoyed marital relations regularly, every week. Yes, high in years, but young and youthful.

Finally, here is the biblical report of the youthfulness of the greatest, most remarkable man who ever lived on this earth, except Jesus Christ, the son of God: "And there arose not a prophet since in Israel like unto Moses, whom the LORD knew face to face" (Deut. 34:10).

Moses' greatness lay in his personality, physical, mental, and spiritual. His extraordinary and noble pilgrimage came to an end at the mountaintop of Horeb. God himself took the honor of his servant into his own keeping, burial and resurrection. The obituary we find recorded in Deuteronomy 34:7 reads as follows: "And Moses was a hundred and twenty years old when he died: his eye was not dim, nor his natural force abated."

Dr. H. D. M. Spencer puts it this way: "Moses had reached the age of one hundred and twenty years, his eye had not become dim, nor were the juices of his body dried."

The Hebrew word so rendered occurs only here. The proper meaning is "freshness," and is used here of the natural juices of the body. Moses died at the age of 120, young and youthful with freshness.

I have presented these stories here, knowing that the average human being today is unlike Moses, but that his natural forces are only 50 per cent active. Through our study, we now know that something can be done about it, and personality engineering is meant to do it. If you are young, by all means strive to keep your youthfulness. If you have grown old, learn to become young again. It is possible! Keeping young and rejuvenated is an art that can be learned. In these chapters on personality engineering, you will find many roadmarks pointing to this end. Watch for them carefully, follow them faithfully, and you will become a personality, perhaps high in years but young in heart.

> Young are those who can laugh through their tears,
> And can smile in the midst of a sigh—
> And can mingle their youth with their years,
> On the road to the sweet by and by.

SELECTED BIBLIOGRAPHY

Abt, W. L., Ph.D. *The Kye*. Hollywood, Calif.: The Author, 1958.

Brown, Arthur I., M.D. *God and You*. Findley, Ohio: Dunham Publishing Co., 1946.

——, *God's Masterpiece*. Findley, Ohio: Dunham Publishing Co., 1946.

Carqué, Otto and Lilian. *Vital Facts About Foods*. Los Angeles: Natural Brands Inc., 1933.

Davies, Dr. Glen. *Divine Diet*. Hollywood, Calif.: The Author, 1950.

Davis, Adelle. *Let's Eat Right to Keep Fit*. New York: Harcourt, Brace & World, 1954.

DeSeblo, Dr. Leon. *Supreme Law for Prolongation of Life*. Mokelumne Hill, Calif.: Health Research.

Elliott, J. C. *New Health Conscience*. Los Angeles, 1915.

Empringham, James, Sc.D. *Intestinal Gardening*. Los Angeles: Health Educational Society, 1934.

Garten, M. O. *The Cycle of Health*. San Francisco, 1946.

Herald of Health magazine. San Francisco.

Hill, Wilfried. *Prolong Your Health*. London: Health for All Publ. Co., 1949.

Journal for Natural Living magazine. Coalmont, Tenn.

Kirschner, H. E., M.D., and Herbert C. White. *Are You What You Eat?* La Sierra, Calif.: Herbert White Publications, 1960.

Listen magazine. Washington, D.C.

Millard, Nellie D., R.N., and Barry G. King, Ph.D. *Human Anatomy and Physiology*. Philadelphia & London: W. B. Saunders Co., 1954.

Nature's Path magazine. New York.

Prevention magazine. Emmaus, Pa.

Richardson, M. G. *The Diet System.* Washington, D.C.: Washington College Press, 1947.

Risley, E. H., M.D., and H. M. Walton. *Clinical Dietetics.* Mountain View, Calif.: Pacific Press Publ. Assn., 1927.

Tilden, J. H., M.D. *Toxemia Explained.* Mokelumne Hill, Calif.: Health Research.

Walker, N. W., Ph.D., Sc.D. *Are You Slipping?* Phoenix, Ariz.: Norwalk Press, 1961.

------. *Becoming Younger.* Phoenix, Ariz.: Norwalk Press, 1949.

------. *Diet and Salad Suggestions.* Phoenix, Ariz.: Norwalk Press, 1956.

------. *Raw Vegetable Juices.* Phoenix, Ariz.: Norwalk Press, 1955.

White, E. G. *Fundamentals of Christian Education.* Nashville, Tenn.: Southern Publ. Assn., 1923.

------. *Healthful Living.* Battle Creek, Mich.: Medical Missionary Board, 1898.

------. *The Ministry of Healing.* Mountain View, Calif.: Pacific Press Publ. Assn., 1909.

White, Julius Gilbert. *Abundant Health.* Madison College, Tenn.: Julius Gilbert White Bookery, 1944.

In addition there are many magazine articles in *Herald of Health, Journal of Natural Living, Listen, Prevention*, and others by Dr. E. M. Abrahamson, William Drees, Dr. P. H. God-dard, Dr. J. A. Goodfellow, Dr. Andrew Ivy, Dr. A. C. Jordan, Ann Landers, Dr. Victor H. Lindlar, Margaret Neel, Dr. A. W. Pezet, Dr. Michael Rabben, Dr. J. I. Rodale, Evelyn Scott, Thomas M. Steger, Dr. R. T. Trail, Dr. Adolphus van Hohensee, and Dr. M. K. Yerkin.